Study Guide

The Culinary Professional

Instructor's Annotated Study Guide

Second Edition

Joan E. Lewis
Instructional Materials Author
Bloomington, Indiana

Text by
John Draz, CEC, CCE
Christopher Koetke, MBA, CEC, CCE, HAAC

Publisher
The Goodheart-Willcox Company, Inc.
Tinley Park, Illinois
www.g-w.com

Introduction

The *Study Guide* is designed for use with the text *The Culinary Professional.* As you complete the activities in this study guide, you review the vocabulary, techniques, tools, and ingredients presented in the text. There are also activities to reinforce the math skills that will help you succeed in the culinary field.

The activities in this study guide are divided into chapters that correspond to those in the text. By reading the text first, you will have the information needed to complete the activities. Try to complete them without referring to the text. Later, you can check the text to complete any answer you did not finish. At that time, you can also compare your answers to the information in the text.

Manufactured in the United States of America.

ISBN 978-1-61960-260-1

1 2 3 4 5 6 7 8 9 10 – 14 – 19 18 17 16 15 14 13

Instructor's Annotated Study Guide

ISBN 978-1-61960-261-8

1 2 3 4 5 6 7 8 9 10 – 14 – 19 18 17 16 15 14 13

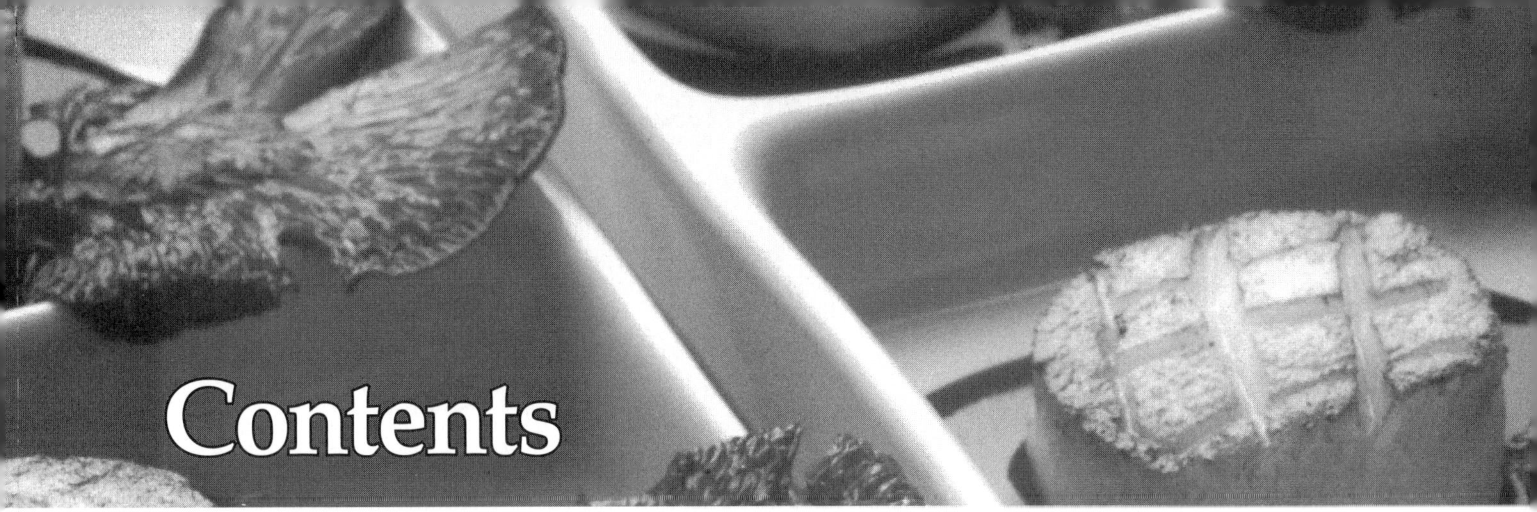

Contents

Welcome to the Foodservice Industry

1

Terminology

Chapter 1 **Name** ______________________

Activity A **Date** __________ **Period** __________

Match the following terms and identifying phrases.

I	1. New practices or conditions that point to the way things will be in the future.	A. cuisine
D	2. The business of making and serving prepared food and drink.	B. culinarian
C	3. Refers to matters related to the preparation or cooking of food.	C. culinary
H	4. Products and practices that can be produced or carried out over a long period of time without a negative effect on the environment.	D. foodservice
F	5. Welcoming guests and satisfying their needs.	E. home meal replacement
A	6. The French word for "kitchen." In the English language, it means a style of cooking.	F. hospitality
E	7. Meals that are consumed at home but professionally prepared elsewhere.	G. living wage
G	8. Rate of pay that allows someone working full-time to support his or her family above the poverty level.	H. sustainable products and practices
B	9. A term for a cook or someone who prepares food.	I. trends

Using Math to Define the Foodservice Industry

Chapter 1 Name ____________________

Activity B Date __________ Period __________

The foodservice industry is so large that it is difficult to grasp. One way to better understand its scope is to think of some of its descriptive statistics in mathematical terms.

A. Estimating output

When you know quantity of output for one time period, you can estimate quantity of output for another time period by multiplication or division. For example, if you know the rate of output for one hour, you could estimate output for an 8-hour day by multiplying the hourly rate by 8. Use this math principle to answer problems 1–3 about the following statistic:

The National Restaurant Association reports that foodservice operations sell over $1.7 billion in meals, snacks, and beverages each day.

1. Estimate the amount of dollars in sales that foodservice operations generate per week.

   $1.7 billion per day x 7 days per week = $11.9 billion in sales per week

2. Estimate the amount of dollars in sales that foodservice operations generate per month (consider a month to be 30 days).

   $1.7 billion per day x 30 days per month = $51 billion in sales per month

3. Estimate the amount of dollars in sales that foodservice operations generate per year.

   $1.7 billion per day x 365 days per year = $620.5 billion per year

B. Graphing statistics

4. One way to get a clearer picture of what statistics are describing is to create a graph. In the space to the right, create a circle graph to show that 27 percent of adults had their first work experience in restaurants. Be sure to label the parts of your graph.

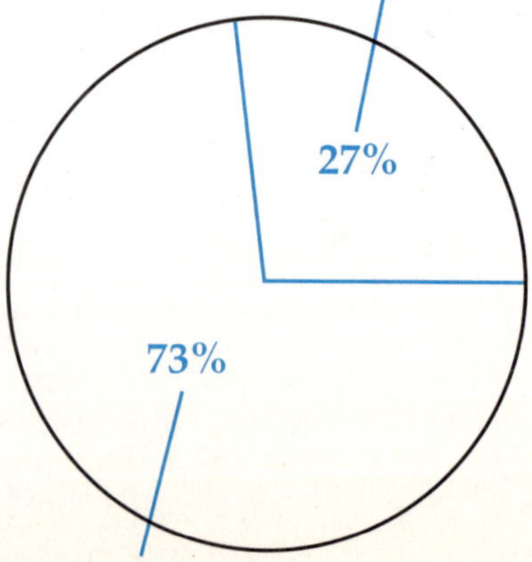

(Continued)

Activity B ***(Continued)*** **Name** ____________________

C. Calculating percent change

Calculating the percent increase or decrease offers another way to evaluate data. To calculate percent increase or decrease, follow these steps:

Step 1. Calculate the difference between the two amounts.

Step 2. Identify the original amount.

Step 3. Substitute these numeric values into this formula: difference ÷ original = decimal

Step 4. Multiply the decimal by 100 and add percent sign.

Example: The number of customers increased from 20 to 25. What was the percent increase in customers?

Step 1. Difference is 25 – 20 = 5

Step 2. Original amount is 20

Step 3. 5 ÷ 20 = 0.25

Step 4. 0.25 x 100 = 25% increase in customers

5. The foodservice industry is projected to grow from 12.9 to nearly 14.3 million employees by 2022. Calculate the percent increase. **14.3 million – 12.9 million = 1.4 million; 1.4 million ÷ 12.9 million = 0.1085; 0.1085 x 100 = 10.85% increase**

Reviewing Key Concepts

Chapter 1 Name ____________________

Activity C Date __________ Period __________

Part 1: Trends in Foodservice

Read the following descriptions of current trends in foodservice. Complete each paragraph by writing the foodservice trend to which the paragraph refers on the space provided.

1. Through travel and the media, diners are more and more exposed to an ever-widening array of dishes from around the world. Restaurateurs and chefs are constantly exploring the world of food for new items to put on their menus. These practices help promote the
 __global__ __cuisine__.

2. Foodservice professionals must be able to use spreadsheets and word processing because these are essential tools for management and communications. Advances in cooking equipment allow food to be cooked faster and better than before. New kitchen equipment is making dramatic changes in the way work is done. These developments are bringing about support for more
 __technological__ __developments__.

3. The foodservice industry is concerned about the environment. There is a growing interest in utilizing products and practices that can be produced or carried out over a long period of time without a negative effect on the environment. These interests encourage the use of
 __sustainable__ __products__ __and__ __practices__.

4. More people are working outside the home and working longer hours. Busy lifestyles leave many people with no time to prepare their own food. These changes are supporting the increase in number of foodservice operations that offer
 __home__ __meal__ __replacement__.

Part 2: Challenges to the Foodservice Industry

Recognizing challenges is the first step in finding solutions. Check each of the following statements that are currently considered challenges for the foodservice industry.

______ 5. Creating enough jobs to supply all the trained workers.

__✓__ 6. Finding enough trained workers to fill all the jobs.

__✓__ 7. Finding ways to pay higher wages and still meet customers' demands for lower prices.

______ 8. Finding ways to lower the minimum wage established by federal law.

__✓__ 9. Meeting the demands for healthier menu options.

__✓__ 10. Producing food that is both satisfying and healthy.

__✓__ 11. Determining chefs' and restaurateurs' responsibility for the health of their guests.

(Continued)

Activity C *(Continued)* **Name** ______________________

Part 3: The Culinary Profession

Read each statement below. Circle the letter *T* if the statement is true. If the statement is false, circle *F* and write the corrected statement on the lines that follow.

(T) F 12. The essential mission for culinarians is to prepare safe and satisfying food for guests.

____

____

T (F) 13. People who typically seek to improve and grow find the culinary profession boring.

Culinarians always have something new to taste and learn.

____

T (F) 14. It is necessary for chefs to know how to prepare food from all cuisines.

No one can know all there is to know about food and cooking. Chefs often specialize in a particular cuisine.

____

(T) F 15. The job of a culinary professional comes with great physical demands.

____

____

T (F) 16. Hours of work for culinary jobs are typically short because the work is centered on mealtimes.

This field often requires working long hours, nights, weekends, and holidays.

Notes

Understanding Foodservice Operations

2

Terminology

Chapter 2 Name ______________________________

Activity A Date ____________ Period ____________

Circle the clue in parentheses that best completes each of the following statements.

1. The term (**full-service restaurant**) (**chain restaurant**) (**franchise restaurant**) refers to a restaurant that is part of a group of restaurants owned by the same company.
2. A (**full-service restaurant**) (**chain restaurant**) (**franchise restaurant**) is characterized by employing servers to take the customers' orders and bring the meals to their tables.
3. A business in which only one person owns and often operates the business is a (**partnership**) (**sole proprietorship**) (**franchise**).
4. Catering is (**providing food and service for groups**) (**operating the business on your own**) (**being part of a large company**).
5. A (**partnership**) (**corporation**) (**sole proprietorship**) is granted a charter from the state, which recognizes it as a separate entity with legal rights.
6. An entrepreneur is (**a business in which one person owns and often operates the business**) (**a business with a charter from the state**) (**a person who organizes a business and assumes all the risk for it**).
7. Franchise restaurants are (**operated by one person**) (**part of a larger restaurant chain, but are independently owned**) (**all owned by the same company**).
8. A (**partnership**) (**corporation**) (**sole proprietorship**) is a business in which ownership is shared by two or more people.
9. Quick-service restaurants are some of the (**least reasonable**) (**most lucrative**) (**most successful**) operations in the industry.

Identifying Foodservice Establishment Options

Chapter 2 Name ____________________

Activity B Date __________ Period __________

Complete the organizational chart showing the various types of foodservice establishments that employ chefs and cooks. Fill in each numbered shape with a term or phrase from the following list.

Banquet facilities	Hotels
Business and organization locations	Off-premise catering
Clubs	Banquet facilities for members
Fine dining	Quick service

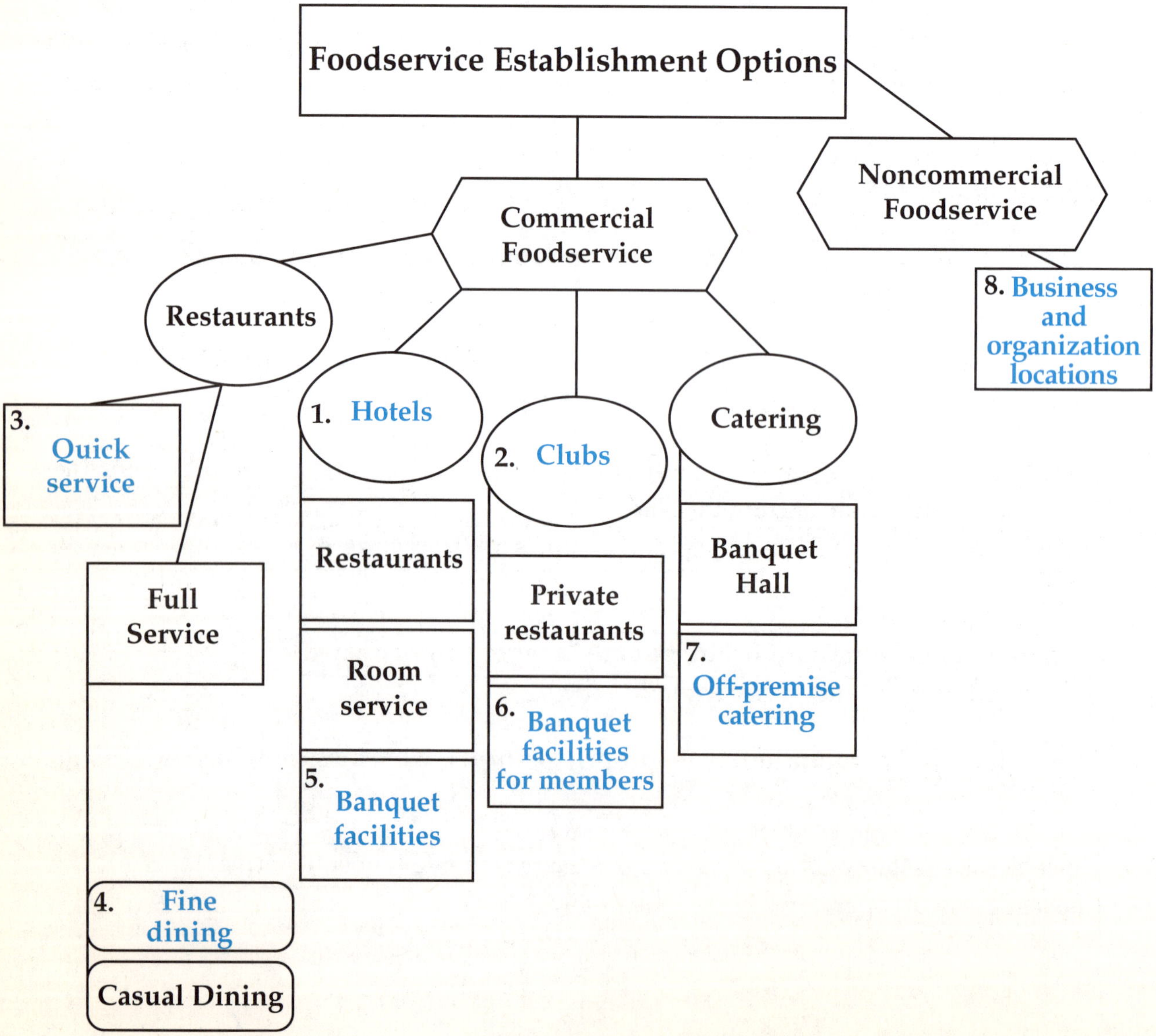

Reviewing Key Concepts

Chapter 2 | **Name** ______________________

Activity C | **Date** __________ **Period** __________

Part 1: Forms of Business Ownership

Foodservice operations, like any business, can take different forms of ownership. The three main legal categories of ownership are ***sole proprietorship, partnership,*** and ***corporation.*** Write the category of ownership that best matches each description.

Description	Category of Ownership
1. A business that is owned equally by three people.	partnership
2. A business that has been granted a charter from the state.	corporation
3. A business that has shareholders who are not responsible for debts of the business.	corporation
4. A business that is owned by one person who also operates the business.	sole proprietorship
5. Legally, this business agreement ends if one of the four owners dies or leaves the business.	partnership
6. In this business, one person has final authority on all decisions.	sole proprietorship
7. A business that has most of the rights and responsibilities of a real person.	corporation
8. This business will continue even if one of the several owners dies or leaves.	corporation
9. The single owner is personally responsible for all debts of this business.	sole proprietorship
10. The two owners of this business are each personally responsible for all the debts of the business.	partnership

(Continued)

Activity C *(Continued)* **Name** ______________________

Part 2: Ways to Organize Foodservice Businesses

Foodservice businesses can be organized in three major ways: independent, chain, and franchise. Various characteristics of foodservice business organizations are listed in this activity. In the space at the left, write ***independent, chain,*** or ***franchise*** to indicate the type of foodservice business organization that is described.

chain 11. Often referred to as "multi-unit foodservice operations."

independent 12. Can quickly adapt to meet the needs of the guests.

chain 13. Their size allows them to buy products more cheaply than a single restaurant.

franchise 14. Are independently owned but part of a large group of restaurants.

franchise 15. The owner pays for the right to use the brand name, concept, logo, and advertising of the original company.

chain 16. Outback Steakhouse restaurant is an example of this type of organization.

franchise 17. McDonald's restaurant is an example of this type of organization.

independent 18. Is a unique operation.

chain 19. Have difficulty implementing changes because there are multiple units.

chain 20. Work hard to make the food and service consistent among all their units.

Part 3: The Risks and Rewards of Entrepreneurship

An entrepreneur is someone who organizes a business and assumes the risk for it. There are risks and rewards of entrepreneurship. Describe the main types of risks and rewards to consider before becoming an entrepreneur.

21. Main type of risk: financial risks

22. Main type of reward: possible financial gain and personal and professional pride

3

Culinary History

Terminology

Chapter 3 | Name ______________________
Activity A | Date __________ Period __________

Match the following terms and identifying statements.

Part 1

B 1. A cuisine that is composed of the best aspects of various cuisines.

H 2. The rebirth that marked the end of the Middle Ages.

D 3. An elaborate, time-consuming style of cooking popular in the early 1800s that was often practiced in the homes of the rich.

F 4. Those foods native to or traditional to a particular geographic region or ethnic population.

A 5. Orderly menus organized by courses that were served tableside by waiters in hotels and restaurants.

E 6. The highest level of the culinary arts in which the most challenging dishes are prepared.

G 7. A style of cuisine that highlighted individual ingredients that were simply prepared and served in small portions on artistic plates.

C 8. The merging of two or more ethnic cuisines into one cooking style.

A. classic cuisine
B. eclectic cuisine
C. fusion cuisine
D. grande cuisine
E. haute cuisine
F. indigenous cuisine
G. nouvelle cuisine
H. Renaissance

Influences on Culinary Practices

Chapter 3 **Name** ______________________

Activity B **Date** __________ **Period** __________

Match the following time periods with the descriptions of developments in culinary practices. Time periods may be used more than once.

__F__ 1. During this period, the Arabs invaded various lands and ruled for hundreds of years. With the invasion of Arabian culture came new cooking techniques and ingredients including almonds, eggplant, citrus fruits, spices, sugar, and rice. Arabs introduced distillation and the addition of sugar and ground nuts to many savory preparations.

__E__ 2. Diets of this era were very different for various classes. While most of the population existed on simple foods prepared in simple ways, the wealthy ate a variety of foods prepared in very complex ways. The chefs of the wealthy were exposed to and learned to use costly imported items such as spices, hams, and oysters.

__A__ 3. The French Revolution caused many chefs who worked in private homes to find themselves without jobs. Necessity gave them a new idea. They opened restaurants. Notably, Antonin Carême wrote books in which he refined and systemized the grande cuisine.

__E__ 4. The first complete Western cookbook was written during this time and was subsequently revised over the next several hundred years. It described challenging culinary dishes with complex flavor profiles and remained the most important cookbook for some time.

__D__ 5. People in this era focused on food products rather than on elaborate cooking techniques. Cooking techniques centered on spit roasting, boiling, baking, and grilling. Foods included olives, honey, cheese, seafood, grain, lamb, and wild herbs.

__B__ 6. A time of rapid technological change. Foods from other countries became readily available and new inventions, such as the microwave, food processor, and convection ovens, changed the way commercial kitchens operated.

A. 1700s and 1800s
B. 1900s
C. Ancient Egypt
D. Ancient Greece
E. Ancient Rome
F. Middle Ages
G. Renaissance

(Continued)

Activity B ***(Continued)*** **Name** ______________________________

C	7. People of this era made yeast-raised and flat breads, tended bees, domesticated animals for milk and meat, and cooked fish.	A. 1700s and 1800s
G	8. During this period, the first voyages to the Americas introduced new products such as tomatoes, potatoes, peppers, corn, and chocolate to Europe.	B. 1900s
F	9. During this era, the Catholic Church, through the efforts of its monasteries, preserved records of ancient cooking practices and preserved and improved the art of baking as well as techniques for making cheese, wine, and beer.	C. Ancient Egypt
G	10. During this period, the marriage of Caterina de Medici to King Henry II of France contributed to the slow and steady refining of French cooking that would lead to the popularity of French cuisine around the world in the centuries that followed.	D. Ancient Greece
		E. Ancient Rome
		F. Middle Ages
		G. Renaissance

Reviewing Key Concepts

Chapter 3 Name ______________

Activity C Date __________ Period __________

Part 1

Read each statement below. Circle the letter *T* if the statement is true. If the statement is false, circle *F* and write the corrected statement on the lines that follow.

(T) F 1. The knowledge chefs learn by studying culinary history gives them a better understanding of the present state of cuisine and where it is headed in the future.

____

____

(T) F 2. The development of agriculture improved standards of living for ancient cultures and resulted in more complex cooking practices.

____

____

T (F) 3. Grande cuisine, refined and systemized in the 1800s, was based on serving simple foods that were simply prepared.

Grande cuisine, refined and systemized in the 1800s, was an elaborate and time-consuming style of cooking.

T (F) 4. Many of the chefs who introduced nouvelle cuisine were influenced by French food traditions.

Many of the chefs who introduced nouvelle cuisine were influenced by Asian food traditions.

(T) F 5. Escoffier simplified grande cuisine by serving fewer, less complicated dishes to create classic cuisine.

____

____

(Continued)

Activity C *(Continued)* **Name** ____________________

T (F) 6. The highest level of the culinary arts where the most challenging dishes are prepared is fusion cuisine.

The highest level of the culinary arts where the most challenging dishes are prepared is haute cuisine.

(T) F 7. Air travel allowed easy contact between chefs in various countries, which has influenced cuisine development.

____

____

Part 2

Complete the flowchart below, which shows the progression of styles of cuisine in sequence by writing one of the following terms in the spaces provided: ***Classic, Fusion, Grande, Nouvelle.***

8. Grande cuisine → 9. Classic cuisine → 10. Nouvelle cuisine → 11. Fusion cuisine

Part 3

Complete the following in the space provided.

12. The television chef star who popularized French cooking in the United States beginning in the 1960s is Julia Child.

13. Name four types of ethnic cuisines other than French that chefs introduced to the American palate beginning in the 1980s.

Thai | Mexican
Cajun | Italian

14. Chefs that mixed different ethnic cuisines to create a new type of cuisine called it fusion cuisine.

(Continued)

Activity C *(Continued)* **Name** ______________________

15. While some chefs were exploring ethnic cuisines, others were creating variations of traditional regional favorites. Name one example of such a dish.

    (List one:) crab cakes, pot roast

16. Explain the term *melting pot cuisine* in relationship to the United States.

    (Answer should include at least the following points:) Waves of new immigrants coming to the United States added their own culinary traditions to those already established. This collection of food traditions was considered something new—a melting pot of cuisines.

Workstations in the Professional Kitchen

4

Brigade Terminology

Chapter 4
Activity A

Name ______________________________
Date ____________ **Period** ____________

Match the following terms and identifying phrases.

Part 1

I 1. Prepares all fish and shellfish items.

G 2. Is in charge of the cold food station. Makes salads, dressing, fruit plates, and other cold preparations.

C 3. The title used for someone who is in charge of a particular workstation in the kitchen.

L 4. Also called the *swing chef* or *roundsman*, this position fills in for other staff members on their days off.

B 5. Cuts and trims meats and poultry for other stations in the kitchen.

H 6. The head of the baking and pastry department who oversees the work of specialists in that station.

E 7. Oversees the preparation and cooking of vegetables, starches, egg dishes, and hot appetizers.

F 8. Reads the servers' food orders to the cooks and organizes the finished dishes so servers can deliver them promptly.

K 9. Is responsible for making sauces.

J 10. Makes all stocks, soups, and mother sauces.

A 11. Makes breads and may also make breakfast pastries.

D 12. Is responsible for preparing meals for the staff in large operations.

A. baker
B. butcher
C. chef de partie
D. communard
E. entremetier
F. expeditor
G. garde manger
H. pastry chef
I. poissonier
J. potager
K. saucier
L. tournant

(Continued)

Activity A *(Continued)* **Name** ____________________

Part 2

A 13. Supervises all the positions in the kitchen, and is responsible for the quality of the food and the safety of the guests and cooks.

E 14. Prepares and cooks deep-fried items.

B 15. The night chef who is in charge of the kitchen after the chef has left for the evening.

J 16. The second in command who assumes the authority and responsibility of the chef when the chef is absent.

D 17. Decorates cakes and pastries and makes chocolate carvings or sugar sculptures for pastry displays.

F 18. Cooks all grilled and broiled meats, poultry, and fish.

H 19. Prepares primarily sweets and pastries.

I 20. In charge of roasting meats and poultry and preparing pan sauces or gravies.

G 21. Prepares and cooks vegetables.

C 22. Assistants in various departments.

A. chef de cuisine
B. chef de garde
C. commis
D. decorator
E. fry cook
F. grill cook
G. légumier
H. pastry cook
I. rotisseur
J. sous chef

Modern Kitchen Organization

Chapter 4 Name ______________________

Activity B Date __________ Period __________

Professional kitchens of a hundred years ago required larger staffs than are needed today. Show your understanding of the factors that influence modern kitchen staff organization by answering the following questions.

1. What three factors contribute to the reduced need for staff in the modern kitchen? Consider operation size, technology, and menu.

   Operations are smaller; modern equipment saves labor time; menus are limited

2. What is the most important factor for determining the staff size and organization of a modern kitchen?

   the menu

3. What is the title of the person hired by hotels or resorts to coordinate the operation of their restaurants and departments?

   executive chef

4. What is the title of the person hired by many hotels to head a special department that prepares meals for large groups?

   banquet chef

5. Traditional kitchens created specialists. When a specialist was absent, it was a problem. How does the modern kitchen use cross training to solve that problem?

   It teaches staff to do more than one job in the kitchen, therefore, other employees will be able to perform the absent person's job.

6. What are three advantages of cross training? Consider scheduling, absenteeism, and job satisfaction.

   Chef has more flexibility in assigning jobs; if a cook is absent, another employee can perform his or her job; work is more interesting if employees don't have to perform the same task every day.

Reviewing Key Concepts

Chapter 4 Name ____________________

Activity C Date __________ Period __________

Part 1: Working with Other Departments

In large foodservice operations, the kitchen works with other departments. Each department has specific responsibilities. Determine which department is responsible for each of the tasks listed. Below, write the letter of each task in the box under the department that is responsible for it.

Departments Beyond the Kitchen				
Catering	**Dining Room**	**Purchasing**	**Room Service**	**Stewarding**
E, F	G	C, D	A	B, H, I, J

Tasks

A. Bring foodservice orders to guests' rooms

B. Clean the kitchen

C. Ensure the right products and correct quantities are being purchased

D. Issue goods and supplies out of the storeroom to the cooks as needed

E. Plan banquets

F. Plan catered events

G. Serve the food

H. Store, inventory, and transport serviceware

I. Warewashing

J. Wash pots and pans

(Continued)

Activity C ***(Continued)*** **Name** ______________________

Part 2: Trends in Foodservice to Reduce Labor

Labor is one of the largest costs in the foodservice industry. Advances in foodservice equipment technology have helped reduce the staff size in commercial kitchens. Explain how each of the following pieces of equipment reduces labor needs in the kitchen.

1. Food processors and grinders: Allows one cook to do the chopping and grinding that would require many cooks to do by hand.
2. Roll-in-rack ovens: Allows one cook to load and remove hundreds of portions from ovens.
3. Machines that vacuum-pack prepared food: Allows one cook to reheat and plate entrées that used to take several cooks to prepare.

Many prepared food products, such as precut vegetables, prepared sauces, and frozen pre-cooked meats and vegetables are used in modern kitchens. These products cost more than the basic ingredients needed to make the item.

4. Why do chefs choose these products? The savings in labor cost is greater than the increased product cost.

Notes

The Professional Chef

5

Terminology

Chapter 5 **Name** ____________________

Activity A **Date** __________ **Period** __________

Match the following terms and identifying statements.

J 1. The supplies, money, or staff that a company needs to do business.

H 2. The positive behaviors and appearance exhibited by an individual who is committed to a career in the culinary arts.

G 3. Composed of or including different elements.

D 4. How you think and feel about other people and situations.

K 5. A physical, mental, and emotional response to external pressures.

F 6. A disagreement with a coworker.

C 7. A method of training in which a person learns a trade under the guidance of skilled tradespeople.

B 8. The largest professional organization for culinarians in the United States.

E 9. Confirmation that a culinarian possesses certain knowledge, skill level, and experience.

A 10. A technique that signals to the speaker that what he or she is saying is understood.

I 11. Nutrition professionals who have completed at minimum a bachelor's degree in dietetics, an internship, and passed a national exam.

A. active listening
B. American Culinary Federation (ACF)
C. apprenticeship
D. attitude
E. certification
F. conflict
G. diversity
H. professionalism
I. registered dietitian (RD)
J. resource
K. stress

What It Takes to Be a Chef

Chapter 5 **Name** ____________________

Activity B **Date** __________ **Period** __________

Part 1: The Roles Chefs Fulfill

To successfully run a commercial kitchen, a chef must fulfill many roles including ***cook, leader, manager, artistic innovator, teacher,*** and ***mentor***. Complete the following statements with the appropriate role.

1. Chefs taking the role of ___artistic innovator___ create new dishes for daily specials and market menus. Occasionally, they create an entirely new menu.
2. Chefs taking the role of ___cook___ judge the quality of food products being prepared by the cooks.
3. Chefs taking the role of ___manager___ manage both people and resources.
4. Chefs taking the role of ___teacher and mentor___ teach the staff cooking skills, management skills, how to deal with people, and more.
5. Chefs taking the role of ___leader___ organize and direct the efforts of the kitchen staff to achieve their version of cuisine.

Part 2: Professional Traits of Successful Culinarians

Professionals are expected to demonstrate the following traits: ***respectful, punctual and dependable, positive attitude, flexible, productive***. For each of the following examples of culinary professional behavior, write the trait being demonstrated.

___productive___ 6. Works efficiently.

___punctual and dependable___ 7. Regularly comes to work on time.

___positive attitude___ 8. Not easily discouraged.

___flexible___ 9. Responds to unexpected events and adjusts plans as needed.

___respectful___ 10. Treats people of all cultures with equal courtesy.

___flexible___ 11. Adapts cooking methods or menu to fluctuations in resources.

___productive___ 12. Balances speed, accuracy, and safety.

Reviewing Key Concepts

Chapter 5 **Name** ____________________

Activity C **Date** __________ **Period** __________

Part 1: Knowledge and Expertise Chefs Must Have

In addition to being an expert cook, a chef must have expertise in several other areas. Match the area of expertise to the example of specific knowledge to which it best relates.

Examples of Specific Knowledge

C 1. The rules and procedures of table service.

G 2. How to interact well with diners and the public at-large.

A 3. Basic mathematics and common bookkeeping procedures.

F 4. The latest information on nutrition.

B 5. How to manage preventive maintenance on appliances.

I 6. Microbiology and basic chemistry of sanitation management.

H 7. How to select, receive, and store the food used in the kitchen.

E 8. The laws that affect the foodservice industry.

D 9. How foods react chemically and physically during the cooking process.

Areas of Expertise

A. cost accounting
B. equipment maintenance
C. food and beverage service
D. food chemistry and physics
E. laws of the foodservice industry
F. nutrition
G. public relations
H. purchasing and storekeeping
I. sanitation

(Continued)

Activity C *(Continued)* **Name** ______________________

Part 2: Education and Training in the Culinary Arts

Match the following terms and identifying phrases.

G 10. Informal training and learning acquired through work experience..

C 11. Are evidence of the evolution of chefs to be regarded as professionals rather than tradespeople.

E 12. Have begun to offer culinary and hospitality training and made the courses career focused.

A 13. Are ways to learn a trade under the guidance of skilled tradespeople.

B 14. Is considered by many to be the standard level of education for culinary management positions.

F 15. Is considered essential for all culinary professionals because of the dynamic conditions of the field.

D 16. Internships and work-based experience are part of the programs offered here.

A. apprenticeships
B. associate's degree
C. bachelor's and advanced degrees in culinary arts
D. career tech and technical high schools
E. high schools
F. lifelong learning
G. on-the-job training

Part 3: Allied Professions

In addition to a career as a chef, Chapter 5 discusses many other professional options in foodservice. These professions require knowledge and skills similar to those of a chef. Next to each of the following statements, write one of the professions discussed in Chapter 5 that best matches the stated preference or interest.

food writer 17. Likes to write about food.

culinary instructor 18. Has the ability to teach.

registered dietitian 19. Wants to help increase the public's food knowledge and culinary skill to improve nutrition and health status.

marketing and sales 20. Interested in selling and promoting.

research chef 21. Interested in working in a manufacturing plant rather than a restaurant kitchen.

personal chef 22. Wants to cook for just one family.

restaurant consultant 23. Wants to advise other professionals.

Entering the Workforce

6

Terminology

Chapter 6 **Name** ______________________

Activity A **Date** __________ **Period** __________

Match the following terms and identifying statements.

I	1. A person who knows and can discuss your work history and personal qualities.	A. benefits
F	2. Opportunity to receive instruction on specific skills or procedures of the job while working.	B. cover message
K	3. Any unwelcome sexual advance, request for sexual favor, and other verbal or physical conduct of a sexual nature that affects a person's ability to work.	C. Equal Employment Opportunity Commission (EEOC)
B	4. A formal business letter or e-mail that introduces a candidate to a potential employer.	D. Fair Labor Standards Act (FLSA)
D	5. Act passed in 1938 to protect workers from unfair treatment by employers.	E. minimum wage
M	6. Refers to valuing and respecting the contributions of coworkers who are different from you.	F. on-the-job training
A	7. Non-wage, financial extras provided by employers to their employees.	G. probation period
L	8. How you feel about your job and how much effort you put into it.	H. progressive discipline
C	9. US agency responsible for the oversight and coordination of all federal equal opportunity regulations, practices, and policies.	I. reference
J	10. A summary of the important information about an applicant.	J. résumé
E	11. The lowest hourly rate of pay that an employee can be paid legally.	K. sexual harassment
G	12. A length of time during which the supervisor observes a new employee to see if he or she is able to perform the job.	L. work ethic
H	13. A method for dealing with unacceptable job-related behavior in a step process.	M. workplace diversity

Reviewing Key Concepts

Chapter 6 **Name** ______________________

Activity B **Date** __________ **Period** __________

Part 1: The Search for Job Opportunities

Circle the clue in parentheses that best completes each of the following statements.

1. You can improve your life and your career opportunities by (**identifying jobs**) (**setting goals**).
2. A parent or other relative (**can**) (**cannot**) be a job-search contact.
3. An acceptable reference is your (**coach**) (**relative**) (**coach or relative**).
4. A good résumé is (**long and detailed**) (**short and concise**).
5. You should find three adults that agree to serve as references (**when you are asked for references at an interview**) (**before beginning your job search**).
6. A work history (**should**) (**should not**) include internships and volunteer positions.
7. Mentioning awards, licenses, and certificates on a résumé is (**appropriate**) (**not appropriate**).
8. You (**should**) (**should not**) list languages spoken on your résumé.
9. Communicating with your job-search contacts to let them know you are looking for a job is called (**work ethic**) (**networking**).
10. List four possible sources of information on job opportunities that you could use to find jobs.

    job-search contacts, school career counselors, professional publications, potential employers, the Internet

Part 2: Submitting Your Résumé

Read each statement below. Circle the letter *T* if the statement is true. If the statement is false, circle *F* and write the corrected statement on the lines that follow.

T F 11. Once you identify a job opportunity, you should submit your résumé promptly.

____

____

(Continued)

Activity B *(Continued)* **Name** ______________________

T F 12. A résumé is a primary tool for getting an interview with a potential employer.

____

____

T F 13. A résumé that is used on the Internet is usually referred to as a computer résumé.

A résumé that is used on the Internet is usually referred to as an electronic résumé.

T F 14. Cover messages are always optional.

Cover messages should always accompany résumés.

____

T F 15. A good cover message is long, detailed, and provides full background, as well as your future plans and desires.

A good cover message is short and to the point.

____

Part 3: The Job Application

Circle the clue in parentheses that best completes each of the following statements.

16. It is (**important**) (**unnecessary**) to bring more information than your résumé when applying for a job because job applications (**often**) (**rarely**) request additional information.
17. Hiring managers typically review the prospective employee's (**résumé rather than job application**) (**job application rather than résumé**) (**résumé and job application**).
18. A portfolio is a selection of materials that prove (**you are trustworthy**) (**your qualifications**).
19. When filling out a job application, neatness (**is**) (**is not**) important.
20. Completing a job application online or at a computer terminal (**allows employers to screen applicants for basic computer skills**) (**allow many more people to apply**).
21. Questions left unanswered (**are not important**) (**raise concerns**).
22. Your answers to questions on a job application (**must match**) (**typically vary slightly from**) the information given on your résumé.

Reviewing Key Concepts

Chapter 6 Name ____________________

Activity C Date __________ Period __________

Part 1: Effective Job Interviews

Complete the following statements describing ways to be effective during the job interview.

1. Prepare for the interview by learning enough about the employer to discuss why you want to work there.
2. Dress appropriately by looking clean, well groomed, and professional.
3. Introduce yourself with a smile and firm handshake.
4. Answer the interviewer's questions as specifically as possible and provide examples when you can.
5. Ask questions that are positive.

Part 2: Expectations

6. List five expectations that employers have of their employees.
good attendance, punctuality, honesty, cooperation and teamwork, ability to accept criticism

7. List five things that employees can expect their employer to provide.
job description, pay, benefits, work schedules, training and probation periods, policies and procedures

(Continued)

Activity C *(Continued)* **Name** ______________________________

Part 3: Laws of Employment

Circle the clue in parentheses that best completes each of the following statements.

8. There are local, state, and federal laws that (**employers**) (**employees**) (**employers and employees**) must follow.
9. The (**FLSA**) (**EEOC**) establishes minimum wage, overtime pay, and child labor standards.
10. Employers (**may not be**) (**are always**) required to pay minimum wage to all employees.
11. The employer must pay at least (**1 ½**) (**2**) times the employee's regular rate of pay for all hours worked over (**35**) (**40**) in a workweek.
12. The FLSA does not limit the number of hours in a day or the number of days in a week that an employer may require an employee to work as long as the employee is at least (**16**) (**18**) (**21**) years old.
13. State laws (**may be**) (**cannot be**) stricter than the FLSA regulations.
14. The (**FLSA**) (**EEOC**) is responsible for the oversight and coordination of all federal equal employment opportunity regulations, practices, and policies.
15. Title VII of the Civil Rights Act of 1964 makes it illegal to discriminate against anyone because of race, color, sex, and (**national origin**) (**religion**) (**national origin or religion**).
16. The *Family and Medical Leave Act of 1993 (FMLA)* is a federal law requiring employers with 50 or more employees to (**provide unrestricted leave**) (**provide up to 12 weeks of unpaid, job-protected leave to qualified employees**).
17. A company (**may**) (**may not**) require a preemployment drug screening.
18. A company (**may**) (**may not**) require a criminal background check.
19. A company (**may**) (**may not**) require a credit history check.
20. A company (**may**) (**may not**) require verification of degrees and work experience.
21. A company (**may**) (**may not**) require employment eligibility verification.
22. A company (**may**) (**may not**) require employees to be a minimum age.

Notes

Sanitation Hazards

7

Terminology

Chapter 7 Name ______________________

Activity A Date __________ Period __________

Part 1

Match the following terms and identifying phrases.

J 1. The measure of acidity or alkalinity of a substance.

E 2. Harmful organisms that cause foodborne illness.

L 3. The amount of water available for microbial growth in a product.

A 4. Bacteria that require oxygen.

H 5. Sickness caused by eating unsafe food.

K 6. The creation and practice of clean and healthy food-handling habits.

F 7. The presence of unsafe substances or levels of dangerous microorganisms in food.

C 8. Bacteria that thrive without oxygen.

I 9. An organism that lives in and feeds on the body of another live creature.

M 10. A microscopic fungus that consumes sugar and expels alcohol and carbon dioxide gas.

B 11. A protein that the body interprets as a dangerous substance.

D 12. Single-celled organisms that reproduce by dividing.

G 13. When an allergen is transferred from its food of origin to a food that does not contain the allergen.

A. aerobic bacteria
B. allergen
C. anaerobic bacteria
D. bacteria
E. biological hazard
F. contamination
G. cross-contact
H. foodborne illness
I. parasite
J. pH
K. sanitation
L. water activity (a_w)
M. yeast

(Continued)

Activity A *(Continued)* **Name** ______________

Part 2

F 14. Lists the composition of a chemical product, proper procedures for storage and handling, and what to do in case of an emergency.

J 15. Any foods that require time and temperature control for safety (TCS) to limit the growth of pathogens or the formation of dangerous by-products.

D 16. Illness resulting from ingestion of toxins left behind by bacteria that are poisonous substances harmful to humans.

L 17. Temperature range [41°F–135°F (5°C–57°C)] in which bacteria reproduce rapidly.

A 18. Any chemical that contaminates food.

N 19. A very small organism that invades another cell and causes it to reproduce the organism.

I 20. Solid materials that pose a danger to the consumer when present in food.

K 21. A thick-walled, "supersurvival unit."

B 22. Bacteria that can grow either with or without oxygen.

C 23. Illness resulting from live bacteria.

H 24. An organism that causes illness in humans.

G 25. The name for a large family of single-cell fungi.

M 26. An infection that occurs when bacteria are ingested and then produce harmful toxins while in the human digestive tract.

E 27. How chemicals seep into food and contaminate it.

A. chemical hazard
B. facultative bacteria
C. infection
D. intoxication
E. leach
F material safety data sheets (MSDS)
G. mold
H. pathogen
I. physical hazard
J. potentially hazardous food
K. spore
L. temperature danger zone
M. toxin mediated infection
N. virus

Identifying Hazards

Chapter 7 **Name** ____________________________

Activity B **Date** ___________ **Period** ___________

1. Select the appropriate food terms or procedures from the following list to complete the "Bacteria" chart below. Place the letter from each correct selection in the appropriate box. (Some terms and procedures will not be used.)

A. Limit time in temperature danger zone
B. Dried fruits
C. High protein foods
D. Add alkaline ingredients to food
E. Reduce amount of oxygen available to bacteria
F. Raw seed sprouts
G. Add water to food
H. Remove water from food
I. Cut tomatoes
J. Handle high protein and other potentially hazardous foods with care
K. Add acidic ingredients to food
L. Store food between 41°F and 135°F

Bacteria	
Favored food sources	C, F, I
Ways to control growth	A, E, H, J, K

2. Repeat the steps described above to complete the "Viruses" chart below.

A. Buy food in bulk
B. Purchase food only from reputable suppliers
C. Raw salad ingredients
D. Hard cooked eggs
E. Expose food to open air
F. Raw or undercooked shellfish
G. Wash raw vegetables before eating
H. Practice excellent personal hygiene
I. Add acidic ingredients to food
J. Avoid shellfish harvested from polluted waters

Viruses	
Likely food sources	C, F
Ways to avoid contamination	B, G, H, J

(Continued)

Activity B *(Continued)* **Name** ______________________

3. Review the information in Chapter 7 and complete the remaining charts.

Fungi			
Types that cause food contamination	poisonous wild mushrooms	yeast	mold
Characteristics	Often shares a similar appearance with edible wild mushrooms	Characterized by slime, discoloration, bubbles, and an alcoholic or "off" smell	Make food unappealing, but some produce dangerous toxins

Parasites		
Type of Parasite	**Common Food Source(s)**	**How to Prevent Transmission**
Trichinella spiralis	undercooked, infested pork some improperly cooked game meats such as bear	cook whole cuts of pork to an internal temperature of 145°F(63°C) cook whole cuts and ground game to an internal temperature of 160°F(71°C)
Anisakis, and certain varieties of *cestodes* and *trematodes*	raw fish	cook fish to an internal temperature of 140°F(60°C) or freeze fish at -31°F(-35°C) for 15 hours or freeze fish at -4°F(-20°C) for seven days

Fish Toxins		
Toxin	Ciguatera	Scombroid
Fish commonly associated with toxin	red snapper	yellowfin tuna
	grouper	skipjack
	barracuda	bonito
		mackerel

Reviewing Key Concepts

Chapter 7 **Name** ______________________

Activity C **Date** __________ **Period** __________

Part 1: Working with Food Safely

Read each statement below. Circle the letter *T* if the statement is true. If the statement is false, circle *F* and write the corrected statement on the lines that follow.

(T) F 1. Improper food handling can result in foodborne illness.

____

____

T (F) 2. Foodborne illness is inconvenient but never serious.

Foodborne illness can result in permanent injury or death.

____

(T) F 3. Outbreaks of foodborne illness can result in employees being fired.

____

____

T (F) 4. Businesses are not at risk of being sued by customers who contract foodborne illness.

Businesses are at risk of being sued by customers who contract

foodborne illness.

T (F) 5. Serving food that is free of contamination is a goal and responsibility for management alone.

Serving food that is free of contamination must be the goal of all

foodservice workers.

(Continued)

Activity C *(Continued)* **Name** ______________________

Part 2: Classifying Food Safety Hazards

Food contamination can result from biological, chemical, or physical hazards. Classify the following contaminants by checking (✓) the correct column for each.

Contaminant	Types of Food Safety Hazards		
	Biological	Chemical	Physical
Bacteria	✓		
Bleach		✓	
Cleaning supplies		✓	
Fish toxins	✓		
Fungi	✓		
Galvanized steel cookware		✓	
Glass			✓
Grease cutters		✓	
Herbicides		✓	
Insecticides		✓	
Metal shards			✓
Mold	✓		
Parasites	✓		
Pesticides		✓	
Polishes		✓	
Staples			✓
Toothpicks			✓
Viruses	✓		
Zinc		✓	

(Continued)

Activity C *(Continued)* **Name** ____________________

Part 3: Preventing Chemical and Physical Hazards

Use terms from the following list to fill in the missing blanks in the statements below.

chemicals	manufacturer's	separate from
chewed	metal	spices
clearly marked	mix	staples
close to	MSDS	supervisor
dispose	original	thrown out
high	react	
ingestion	seen	

6. Store chemicals in ___clearly___ ___marked___ containers or leave them in their ___original___ package.
7. Do not store food in containers that previously held ___chemicals___.
8. Only use chemicals according to the ___manufacturer's___ instructions.
9. Store chemicals in an area ___separate___ ___from___ food preparation areas.
10. Never randomly ___mix___ chemicals because certain chemicals can ___react___ to create highly poisonous substances.
11. ___Dispose___ of chemicals in accordance with manufacturer's directions.
12. If uncertain about how to use a chemical product, ask a ___supervisor___.
13. In the event of ___ingestion___, call a poison control hotline immediately.
14. Display ___MSDS___ sheets in a visible and accessible place in the kitchen.
15. Do not store glass in ___high___ places. All food that might possibly be contaminated with glass should be ___thrown___ ___out___.
16. When breaking down boxes, be careful that ___staples___ do not enter food.
17. Check contents of cans opened by commercial can openers for ___metal___ shards.
18. When using toothpicks, be sure to use ones that are easily ___seen___.

(Continued)

Activity C *(Continued)* **Name** ______________________

Part 4: Food Allergens

Read each statement below. Circle the letter *T* if the statement is true. If the statement is false, circle *F* and write the corrected statement on the lines that follow.

T (F) 19. An allergy occurs when the body interprets a harmful protein as a physical hazard.

An allergy occurs when the body interprets a normally harmless protein as a dangerous substance.

(T) F 20. Allergic reactions can range from skin irritations to difficulty breathing to death.

T (F) 21. Chefs and cooks are the only staff members that need to treat food allergies seriously.

Everyone in foodservice needs to treat food allergies seriously.

T (F) 22. If a customer tells the waitstaff she is allergic to peanuts, the cooks must avoid most peanut-based ingredients.

If a customer tells the wait staff she is allergic to peanuts, the cooks must avoid all peanuts and peanut-based ingredients.

(T) F 23. All utensils previously used with peanut ingredients must be thoroughly cleaned.

T (F) 24. Cross-contamination occurs when an allergen is transferred from its food of origin to a food that does not contain the allergen.

Cross-contact **occurs when an allergen is transferred from its food of origin to a food that does not contain the allergen.**

(T) F 25. Common sources of allergens include, but are not limited to, dairy products, fish, shellfish, peanuts and peanut products, and tree nuts.

Sanitation Procedures

8

Terminology

Chapter 8 **Name** ____________________

Activity A **Date** __________ **Period** __________

Complete the following statements about sanitation procedures. Then arrange the circled letters to solve problem 9.

1. Any surface such as a table, cutting board, or piece of equipment that comes in contact with food is considered a food-contact surface.
2. A sanitary environment is free from pathogens.
3. A pest control operator is a licensed professional who uses various chemicals, sprays, and traps to prevent or eliminate infestations.
4. A step in food handling at which control can be applied to prevent or eliminate a food safety hazard is a critical control point.
5. Cross-contamination occurs when harmful microorganisms are transferred from one product to another by hands, utensils, equipment, or other physical contact.
6. A three compartment sink consists of three adjacent sinks used to clean, rinse, and sanitize small equipment and utensils.
7. Hazard analysis critical control point is a system that identifies and manages key steps in food handling where contamination is most likely to occur.
8. Clean is the visual appearance that something is unsoiled.

Circled letters: ____________________

9. A key principle to food safety is time and temperature.

Reviewing Key Concepts

Chapter 8 | **Name** ____________________

Activity B | **Date** __________ **Period** __________

Part 1: Time and Temperature

Circle the clue in parentheses that best completes each of the following statements.

1. To protect food from contamination, you must make sure food is (**above**) (**below**) (**above or below**) the temperature danger zone.
2. When food must be in the temperature danger zone, limit the time to no more than (**twelve**) (**eight**) (**four**) (**two**) hours.
3. Thaw frozen food in the refrigerator or under (**hot**) (**warm**) (**cold**) running water.
4. To kill biological hazards present in most foods, cook to an (**internal**) (**external**) (**approximate**) temperature of 145°F (63°C).
5. Food held hot must maintain an (**internal**) (**external**) (**approximate**) temperature of (**145°F [63°C]**) (**135°F [57°C]**) or more.
6. Hot, fully cooked food must be cooled (**slowly**) (**rapidly**).

Part 2: Cross-Contamination

Read the following scenarios. In the space provided, explain where the cross-contamination could occur and how it could be avoided.

7. A cook is assembling cold sandwich plates for a luncheon. A coworker invites him to sign a "get well" card for a sick employee. The cook stops what he is doing, borrows the pen from the coworker, and signs the card. The cook returns to preparing his plates. Cross-contamination occurs when the cook holds the pen and then resumes preparing food. The worker should have washed his hands after handling the pen and before returning to work.

8. A cook cleans and sanitizes her work counter before beginning her assignment. A coworker comes by and asks to borrow a knife. The cook grabs her toolbox and places it on the counter. She finds the knife in her toolbox and loans it to her coworker. She returns her toolbox to its storage place and proceeds with food preparation on her work counter. Cross-contamination occurs when the toolbox is placed on the counter and then the cook resumes preparing food on the counter. The worker should either have kept the toolbox off the counter or cleaned and sanitized the counter after the toolbox was removed and before food preparation resumed.

(Continued)

Activity B ***(Continued)*** **Name** ______________________

9. A cook seasons some raw chicken breasts and lays them out on a sheet pan. He stores the chicken in the refrigerator until he is ready to cook them. The cook places the pan of chicken on the top shelf in the refrigerator because the shelves below are filled with dessert parfaits for a luncheon. **Cross-contamination can occur from the raw chicken breasts dripping into the ready-to-eat desserts. The worker should have moved the bottom tray of desserts to the top shelf and then placed the chicken breast on the bottom shelf and stored them in a leak-proof container.**

Part 3: Cleaning and Sanitizing

10. Explain the following statement: "A kitchen can look clean and still be unsanitary." **Clean is the visual appearance that nothing is soiled. Sanitary refers to an environment that is free from pathogens. Since pathogens are often not visible to the naked eye, a surface could look clean but be contaminated with pathogens.**

For each of the following cleaning and sanitizing techniques, indicate the order in which these steps must be performed. In the space provided, assign each step a number to indicate its order in the sequence. The first step is assigned the number "1" and so on.

Technique for Sanitizing a Counter or Worktable	
Sequence of Steps	**Steps**
3	Rinse table using hot water and a clean towel.
2	Wash the table with hot water and detergent.
5	Allow to air-dry.
1	Clear table or countertop.
4	Apply sanitizer using either a spray bottle or a special sanitizing bucket.

Technique for Using a Dishmachine	
Sequence of Steps	**Steps**
2	Remove visible pieces of food before placing items into machine.
4	Load the rack into the dishmachine.
1	Presoak flatware to loosen encrusted food.
5	When the cleaning and sanitizing cycles are complete, remove from the dishmachine and allow items to air-dry.
3	Place the items to be washed in the appropriate dish rack.

(Continued)

Activity B *(Continued)* **Name** ______________________

Technique for Cleaning and Sanitizing Large Equipment	
Sequence of Steps	**Steps**
7	Sanitize using a sanitizing solution. Follow manufacturer's instructions to determine dilution.
6	Dry using a clean towel or paper towels.
1	Unplug electrical equipment before beginning to clean.
3	Disassemble equipment as needed. Clean and sanitize small parts in a dishmachine or three-compartment sink.
2	Wear cut-resistant gloves if washing a sharp piece of machinery.
5	Rinse with hot water.
4	Wash with hot water and detergent to remove visible grime and pieces of food.

Reviewing Key Concepts

Chapter 8 **Name** ____________________

Activity C **Date** __________ **Period** __________

Part 1: Personal Hygiene

Select the term or phrase from the following list that best completes each statement below. (Some terms will be used more than once.)

20	elbows	six
40	every	soap
air dryer	four	sweat
backs	gloved	under
change	hot	warm
comfortable	paper towel	
communal	roll up sleeves	

A. Technique for proper hand washing

1. Use water that is as hot as is ___comfortable___,at least 110°F (43°C).
2. ___Roll up sleeves___ and wet your hands.
3. Add soap and lather hands, including the ___backs___ and wrists, and up to the ___elbows___. Scrub for ___20___ seconds and use a nailbrush to scrub ___under___ the fingernails. Wash well between fingers.
4. Rinse under ___hot___, running water.
5. Dry using ___paper towel___ or ___air dryer___. Do not dry hands on a ___communal___ towel or apron.
6. Use ___paper towel___ to turn water off and open bathroom door, then discard.

B. Guidelines for using disposable gloves

7. Properly wash hands using ___soap___ before putting on a pair of gloves.
8. Change gloves if ___sweat___ starts to drip out from under gloves.
9. Change gloves after___every___ work task.
10. If gloves become even slightly torn or punctured, ___change___ them.
11. Change gloves at least every ___four___ hours.
12. Never wash ___gloved___ hands.

(Continued)

Activity C *(Continued)* **Name** ______________________

Part 2: Insect, Rodent, and Waste Control

Answer the following questions in the space provided.

13. Name two ways that insects and rodents spread biological hazards in the kitchen. (Relate to pest droppings and garbage.) Pests deposit pathogens in their droppings.
Pests carry pathogens on their bodies and feet from the garbage to the kitchen.

14. What is the most important step in pest control? To keep a clean and sanitized facility.

15. What is the minimum frequency for emptying garbage containers in the kitchen? At the end of each workday.

Part 3: Hazard Analysis Critical Control Point and Health Inspection

Complete the following statements in the space provided.

16. The goal of the Hazard Analysis Critical Control Point (HACCP) system is to analyze food-handling procedures in a kitchen in order to reduce the risk of contamination.

17. HACCP pays particular attention to the temperature danger zone and minimum internal temperatures.

18. HACCP plans rely on predetermined critical control points (CCP). CCP is a step in food handling at which control can be applied to prevent or eliminate a food safety hazard.

19. Health inspectors are responsible for protecting the public health.

20. When a health department official inspects a foodservice operation, foodservice workers should answer their questions honestly.

Safety in the Kitchen

9

Terminology

Chapter 9 **Name** ____________________

Activity A **Date** __________ **Period** __________

Under each of the culinary terms that follow is a list of statements. If the statement is accurate, place a check (✓) in the space provided before each statement.

Fire Extinguisher

__✓__ 1. Commercial kitchens are required by law to have them.

______ 2. Are all the same.

__✓__ 3. Are pressurized canisters filled with a substance that puts fires out.

Heat Exhaustion

______ 4. Is more serious than heatstroke.

__✓__ 5. Is a heat-related condition that results when the body loses too much water and salt.

______ 6. Is often brought on by heatstroke.

__✓__ 7. Can be brought on by working at a fast pace in a hot environment.

Heatstroke

__✓__ 8. Is more serious than heat exhaustion.

__✓__ 9. Is a condition in which the body's usual ability to deal with heat stress is lost.

__✓__ 10. Is potentially life threatening and requires immediate medical attention.

__✓__ 11. Can be brought on by heat exhaustion.

Kitchen Hood Fire Suppression System

__✓__ 12. Required by law for commercial kitchens.

______ 13. Is an installed, comprehensive fire fighting system that automatically sounds an alarm when a fire is detected.

__✓__ 14. Is an installed, comprehensive fire fighting system that automatically puts out a fire before it spreads.

Occupational Safety and Health Administration

__✓__ 15. Is commonly known as OSHA.

__✓__ 16. Requires all workplaces to post the Occupational Safety and Health Administration's safety and health poster and a yearly log of injury and illness.

__✓__ 17. Is a government agency that defines and enforces safe working conditions.

(Continued)

Activity A *(Continued)* **Name** ____________________

Cardiopulmonary Resuscitation (CPR)

___✓___ 18. Is a rescue procedure that combines chest compressions with blowing into the victim's mouth.

______ 19. Simulates the lymphatic system.

___✓___ 20. Both the American Heart Association (AHA) and the American Red Cross suggest anyone can use the Hands-Only™ CPR method.

______ 21. Hands-Only™ CPR requires chest compressions at a rate of 50 per minute.

Automated External Defibrillator (AED)

___✓___ 22. Detects the type of heart rhythm and delivers and electric shock if appropriate.

______ 23. Requires much training, so few people can use them

___✓___ 24. Courses in basic CPR provide training on performing CPR and using an AED.

Prudent

___✓___ 25. A prudent behavior is calling 911 if a fire spreads beyond its initial source.

______ 26. Spraying a grease fire in a sauté pan with water is a prudent behavior.

___✓___ 27. Calling the fire department to inspect damage is a prudent action even if foodservice staff members have put out a fire.

______ 28. The most prudent behavior is spraying a wall with a fire extinguisher if a greasy wall catches on fire.

Roles in Creating Workplace Safety

Chapter 9 **Name** ______________________

Activity B **Date** ____________ **Period** ____________

Government, employers, and employees all play a part in creating a safe workplace. Circle the group (or groups) to whom the workplace safety rights and responsibilities listed in the left column applies.

Workplace Safety Rights and Responsibilities	Who Is Responsible? (Circle all that apply)		
Must maintain a safe workplace by law.	government	employers	employees
Must keep accident reports on file permanently for future reference.	government	employers	employees
Ensures that employers train their employees in safe work practices.	government	employers	employees
Can contact OSHA for advice and help.	government	employers	employees
Periodically are given a review of procedures for safety, sanitation, and hazardous materials.	government	employers	employees
Records and keeps files of employee's attendance at training sessions.	government	employers	employees
Along with witnesses, are asked to fill out accident report forms when accidents occur.	government	employers	employees
Are held responsible for all safety information presented during safety training.	government	employers	employees

Dress for Safety

Chapter 9 **Name** ______________________

Activity C **Date** __________ **Period** __________

Complete the following statements that describe the safety features of the professional culinary uniform.

The Chef Jacket…

1. …is white *because* white reflects heat, which helps keep the cook cool.

2. …is long sleeved *because* long sleeves protect the arms from splattering hot grease or the intense heat of a grill.

3. …is double-breasted *because* the double layer protects the chest from the heat of a stove or oven.

The Chef Pants…

4. …are long *because* long pants protect the legs from burns.

The Apron…

5. …is not to be used for wiping hands *because* wiping hands on the apron could be a source of cross-contamination.

6. …is designed to be easily lifted from the body *because* an employee can immediately lift the apron away from the body to minimize burns from hot spills.

(Continued)

Activity C *(Continued)* **Name** ______________________

Footwear...

7. ...ideally has nonslip soles *because* kitchen floors are often slippery
____
____.

8. ...is never open-toed *because* open-toed shoes provide no protection against a falling knife or heavy object
____.

Jewelry

9. Rings, necklaces, earrings, and bracelets should not be worn in the kitchen *because* this type of jewelry can get caught on moving equipment and cause serious injury
____
____.

10. Small pieces of jewelry, such as those used in piercings, should not be worn in the kitchen *because* small pieces of jewelry can fall in food unobserved and become a physical hazard.

Kitchen Injuries

Chapter 9 **Name** ____________________

Activity D **Date** __________ **Period** __________

Select the term or phrase from the following list that best completes the statements about kitchen injuries below. Some terms or phrases will not be used.

announce	downward	read
appropriate	dull	rubber mats
away	eventually	run or push
backpacks	gesture	sharp
catch	greasy	staff
chop	holding	steam
clear	kitchen	stockpots
cold water	leather	upward
cotton rugs	nonslip	warn
comfortably	promptly	wet towel
cutting	protect	
dishwashing	purses	

A. Preventing cuts

1. Practice correct knife ____cutting____ skills.
2. Always carry a knife by your side and pointed ____downward____ .
3. Always ____announce____ when you are carrying a knife to warn others of the danger.
4. Never leave a knife or sharp object in a ____dishwashing____ sink.
5. Never ____gesture____ with a knife.
6. Never try to ____catch____ a falling knife.
7. Use only ____sharp____ knives.
8. Use knives only for ____appropriate____ tasks, never as hammers or can openers.

(Continued)

Activity D (*Continued*) **Name** ____________________

B. Preventing falls

9. Make sure spills are ____promptly____ wiped up.
10. Clean ____greasy____ floors immediately.
11. Do not place items such as ____stockpots____ or cases of food on the floor.
12. No matter how busy you are, do not ____run or push____ in the kitchen.
13. Place removable ____rubber mats____ wherever the floor is slippery.
14. Keep aisles ____clear____ .
15. Wear shoes with ____nonslip____ soles.
16. Put ladders and stools ____away____ after using them.
17. Be aware of such items as ____purses____ or ____backpacks____ that customers place on the floor.

C. Preventing Burns

18. Never use a damp or ____wet towel____ as a hot pad.
19. Be sure that a hot pad is sufficiently thick to properly ____protect____ your hand from a hot pan.
20. Never place a hot pan at a dishwashing station without alerting the dishwashing ____staff____.
21. When carrying a hot pan or liquid through the kitchen, loudly ____warn____ others by saying "HOT!"
22. Never attempt to move anything hot that you cannot ____comfortably____ carry or lift.
23. Avoid contact with ____steam____ when opening the door of a steamer or lifting the lid off a pot of boiling liquid.
24. If a burn causes the skin to redden or blister, place the burned part of the body in ____cold water____.

Fire Safety

Chapter 9 **Name** ______________________

Activity E **Date** __________ **Period** __________

Part 1: Ingredients for Fire

Three ingredients must always be present to produce fire—*fuel, oxygen,* and *heat*. Indicate which of these ingredient(s) is being removed from each of the scenarios below.

1. The chef would not allow newspapers to be left lying around in the kitchen. Which ingredient for fire did the chef want to remove? **fuel**
2. When a sauté pan caught fire, the cook grabbed a cover and placed it on the pan. Which ingredient for fire did the cook want to remove? **oxygen**
3. The chef insisted that spilled grease be wiped off the stove immediately. Which ingredient for fire did the cook want to remove? **fuel**
4. The server extinguished the candle by blowing on it. Which ingredient for fire did the server want to remove? **heat**
5. The culinary worker threw water on a potholder that caught fire. Which ingredients for fire did the cook want to remove? **heat** and **oxygen**

Part 2: Using Fire Extinguishers

Circle the clue in parentheses that best completes each of the following statements.

6. Use a fire extinguisher only if the fire is (**spreading rapidly**) (**localized**).
7. Position yourself with your (**back**) (**face**) toward an exit.
8. (**Take time**) (**Don't take time**) to verify that you have the correct extinguisher for the type of fire.
9. Pull the pin at the (**top**) (**nozzle**) of the fire extinguisher.
10. Aim at the (**top**) (**base**) of the flames.
11. (**Squeeze**) (**Grip**) the trigger.
12. Sweep (**up and down**) (**back and forth**) so the entire base of the fire is covered repeatedly.
13. Continue to spray until the fire is (**diminished**) (**out**).

Sustainability in the Kitchen 10

Terminology

Chapter 10 **Name** ______________

Activity A **Date** __________ **Period** __________

Match the following terms and identifying phrases.

K 1. The adoption of practices that either preserve or improve the condition of Earth for future generations.

F 2. A measure of the amount of energy needed to move food from its point of harvest to its final destination.

B 3. The variety of forms of animal and plant life in a particular area.

G 4. Plants grown from seeds that have been unchanged for several to many generations.

D 5. Products or practices that do not damage the environment.

E 6. Equipment and systems that use less energy to perform work than conventional alternatives.

H 7. A device that reduces the amount of water that comes from a faucet while directing the water stream.

C 8. The process by which some food and other organic matter decay to form a highly fertile growing substance.

A 9. Ability of something to be broken down into harmless products by living things such as worms, insects, and bacteria.

J 10. An item that can be repurposed and kept out of the waste stream.

I 11. The process by which something is reformulated to be used again.

A. biodegradable
B. biodiversity
C. composting
D. ecofriendly
E. energy efficient
F. food miles
G. heirloom variety
H. low-flow aerators
I. recycling
J. reusable
K. sustainability

Sustainability Concepts

Chapter 10 Name ____________________

Activity B Date __________ Period __________

Use the text to complete the chart that follows. Write your answers in the space provided.

TERM	Applies to	DEFINITION
Antibiotic-free	Meat and dairy products	■ An animal that has either never received antibiotics or sufficient time has lapsed for the drugs to clear out of the animal's system. ■ Some animals are given antibiotics to counteract the effects of crowding, stress-inducing conditions, and unnatural diets. ■ Most antibiotics are given to healthy animals. ■ As much as 80%–90% of antibiotics given to animals and humans are passed through the body and into the water system. ■ They interact and can form more antibiotic-resistant strains that pose a risk to both humans and animals.
Biodynamic	Produce	■ A cultivation method that considers the farm to be a living thing, or organism. ■ This method includes the use of fermented manure, minerals, and herbs to enhance soil health. ■ Soil health influences the nutrient content, quality, and flavor of food grown in it. ■ Originally, biodynamic meant that a farm was completely self-contained and everything used on the farm originated there.
Cage-free	Poultry, eggs	■ Often used with "free-range," this means that domestic fowl (chickens, ducks, etc.) are not raised in cages. ■ Is not a legal definition.
Carbon Footprint		■ The amount of climate-changing carbon emissions from a system or activity often referred to as *greenhouse gases.* ■ The foodservice industry accounts for about one-third of all human greenhouse emissions. ■ These emissions are generated during the transport, production, and consumption of food.

(Continued)

Activity B *(Continued)* **Name** ______________________

Free-range	Beef cattle, sheep, goats, pigs, dairy cattle, and particularly poultry	■ The USDA definition meaning that animals have access to the outside.
Genetically Modified Organisms (GMO)	Produce and animals	■ Plants or animals that have had genes introduced, rearranged, or eliminated to make them more resistant to pests and other elements that endanger the crop and reduce yield. ■ The USDA includes plants or animals altered through traditional breeding methods in this definition.
Grass-fed	Cattle, sheep, goats, and bison	■ Grass-fed cattle consume the majority of their nutrients from grass as opposed to grain, soy, or corn. ■ This label does not limit the use of antibiotics, hormones, or pesticides.
Hormone-free	Meat and dairy products	■ Foods are free of hormones given to stimulate growth and milk production. ■ Although the USDA and FDA deem them safe for human consumption, the European considers them a risk to human health.
Organic	All foods	■ Foods with this certification meet the requirements for production and labeling established by the Organic Foods Production Act. ■ These foods must be produced without the use of synthetic fertilizers, sewage sludge, irradiation, and genetic engineering. ■ Only natural products and methods that promote and protect the environment can be used. ■ Products can be labeled either *100 Percent Organic* or *Organic.*
Wild-caught	Seafood	■ Seafood that is harvested in the wild environments of the ocean, lakes, and rivers. ■ There are many harvesting techniques that vary with the type of seafood being harvested. ■ Some protect fish stocks and others destroy them and the ecosystems.

Reviewing Key Concepts

Chapter 10 **Name** ______________________

Activity C **Date** __________ **Period** __________

Part 1: Sustainability in Foodservice

Circle the clue in parentheses that best completes each of the following statements.

1. Addressing sustainability in the foodservice kitchen is **(unimportant to profitability)** **(a guide for making decisions and choices)** **(just another chef task)**.
2. For better understanding of sustainability in food service, it can be divided into the following categories: **(purchasing, energy, water, waste, and social considerations)** **(energy, landfills, global concerns, water, and product choices)** **(transportation, energy, food preparation, and water)**.
3. Sustainability practices in foodservice **(take a great deal of time)** **(are clearly identified and planned)** **(preserve or improve the condition of the Earth)**.
4. Using sustainable business practices makes good business sense because they **(save time during the workday)** **(can improve profitability)** **(allow the chef to use globally available products)**.
5. Customers view restaurants that pursue sustainable objectives **(less favorably)** **(favorably)** **(indifferently)**.

Part 2: Purchasing Food and Nonfood Products

Read each of the following statements about purchasing food and nonfood products. If a statement about sustainable practices for purchasing food and nonfood products is *accurate*, place a check (✓) in the space provided before the statement.

______ 6. When purchasing large amounts of food and nonfood items such as cleaning products, sustainability becomes a decreasingly important factor in purchasing decisions.

______ 7. Practicing sustainability when purchasing food is complex because there are many variables in the ways food is produced and transported.

______ 8. Sustainably produced food often costs less than traditional industrially produced foods.

______ 9. Because a farmer is trying to put less stress on the soil, livestock, and water supply, sustainable foods may require more labor or produce lower yields.

______ 10. Chefs use different strategies to offset the higher prices paid for sustainable food products to maintain profitability.

______ 11. For sustainability purposes, choosing which foods to purchase is simple. The chef just needs to know where the food was raised and how it was harvested.

(Continued)

Activity C *(Continued)* **Name** ____________________

✓ 12. The measure of the amount of energy (not necessarily distance) needed to move food from its point of harvest to its final destination is called *food miles.*

_____ 13. Moving perishable food by airplane consumes less energy than moving the food by train.

✓ 14. Drawbacks to locally sourced foods include inconsistent availability and lower quality than the same foods grown in other parts of the country.

_____ 15. Locally sourced foods are generally fresher than foods sourced further away, but do little to contribute to the local economy.

✓ 16. Biodiversity is the variety of forms of animal and plant life in a particular area.

✓ 17. Heirloom plants are grown from seeds that remain genetically constant and reflect a long heritage.

✓ 18. *Ecofriendly* refers to products or practices that do not damage the environment.

_____ 19. Ecofriendly cleaning products are generally used the same way as conventional cleaning products.

✓ 20. When choosing a laundry service for a restaurant facility, it is important to investigate the sustainability practices and types of cleaning products services use.

✓ 21. When choosing interior elements such as carpeting or wallcoverings for a restaurant, choose items that do not diffuse volatile organic compounds into the air at room temperatures.

_____ 22. Choosing an effective pest control operator (PCO) to prevent pest infestations is more important than the toxicity of chemicals used to control pests.

Part 3: Food Waste Recovery

Examine the *Food Recovery Hierarchy* table that follows. In the space provided, list the EPA strategies for reducing food waste from *Most Preferred (1)* to *Least Preferred (6).*

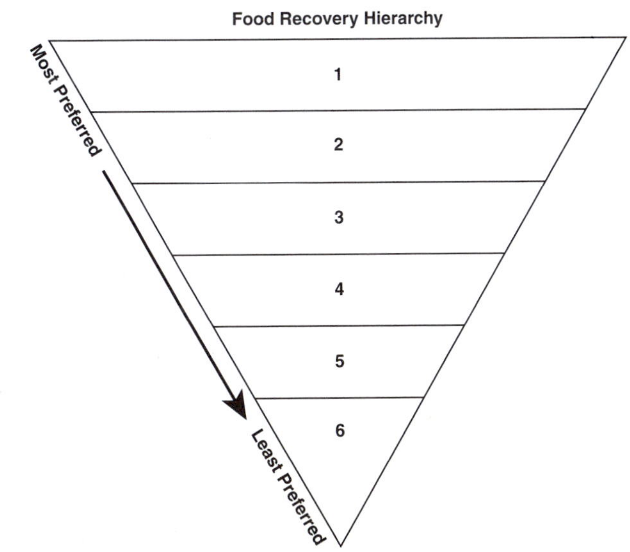

1. Source reduction
2. Feed hungry people
3. Feed animals
4. Industrial uses
5. Composting
6. Incineration or landfill

(Continued)

Activity C *(Continued)* **Name** ______________________

Another way to sustainably address food waste is with *composting*. Complete the chart that follows by identifying two statements that describe each form of composting.

A. Vermicomposting	**(Any two:) Uses worms, along with other bacteria, fungi, and insects to break down the waste into a high-quality fertilizer. This method is typically recommended for food scraps, excluding animal proteins and dairy foods.**
B. Aerobic/Windrow composting	**(Any two:) Exposes the organic matter to bacteria and plenty of oxygen through frequent mixing. The result is the matter gets hot (up to 160°F, 71°C) and breaks down into a rich, fertile substance. This is typically recommended for lawn clippings and leaves. Food scraps, excluding dairy and animal proteins, may be added to the mix.**
C. Anaerobic composting	**(Any two:) This occurs when a large pile of organic matter is simply heaped up and not mixed, as in a landfill. This process: takes longer to break down organic matter and a different kind of bacteria (anaerobic) grows in this oxygen-depleted environment; produces damaging methane gas. While anaerobic composting in a landfill hurts the environment, there are new technologies being employed to produce valuable products instead. These technologies use anaerobic composting in a controlled environment called an anaerobic digester. The anaerobic digester turns food waste into renewable energy and soil amendment by quickly breaking down the materials and capturing the methane gas for use as fuel. The remaining solid materials are added back into soil.**

Part 4: Reuse, Recycle, and Hazardous Waste

Read each statement that follows. Circle the letter *T* if the statement is true. If the statement is false, circle *F* and write the corrected statement on the lines that follow.

(T) F 1. Reuse of waste involves repurposing it to keep it out of the waste stream.

____

____

(Continued)

Activity C *(Continued)* **Name** ____________________

T (F) 2. Plastic film used in the transport of packaging, especially shrink-wrap on pallets received in large operations, is *not* recyclable.

Plastic film used in the transport of packaging, especially shrink-wrap,

is recyclable.

T (F) 3. Most aluminum containers, cans, and foil are recyclable.

Aluminum foil is typically not recyclable due to food residue.

(T) F 4. All forms of glass jars and bottles are recyclable.

T (F) 5. Most paper beverage cups are suitable for recycling.

Most paper beverage cups are unsuitable for recycling.

(T) F 6. Cooking oil can be recycled and turned into a wide variety of products.

T (F) 7. It is best to properly dispose of printer ink cartridges in the trash.

These cartridges can be refilled for reuse or recycled into new plastic.

T (F) 8. Some cities promote disposal of computers and electronic devices in landfills because they are difficult to recycle.

Some cities are banning electronics from landfills.

(T) F 9. It is best to take hazardous waste materials to specific locations capable of disposing these substances in a safe, ecofriendly way.

Sustainability and Social Concerns

Chapter 10 Name ______________________

Activity D Date __________ Period __________

Match the following terms and identifying statements. Terms may be used more than once.

C 1. The culinary community is ideally positioned to set the food fashion that can improve the way people eat.

E 2. Organizations such as Fair Trade USA certify products that meet social sustainability standards.

B 3. When there are people experiencing hunger everyday, there is an obligation to use food resources wisely and thoughtfully.

A 4. A practice of hiring people who are different in ethnicity, gender, gender-orientation, as well as those with disabilities.

D 5. Voicing an opinion is a social responsibility of all citizens.

A 6. Considering differences when hiring, designing work spaces, providing service, or writing menus.

C 7. A threat to the health and welfare of citizens and future generations.

E 8. Placing an importance on the wholesomeness of the food sold and methods used to raise and grow it.

D 9. Staying informed about current topics.

B 10. Foodservice in the United States has taken a leadership role in trying to alleviate hunger

A. Diversity

B. Food waste

C. Obesity

D. Public policy

E. Purchasing

Knives and Hand Tools in the Professional Kitchen

11

Terminology

Chapter 11 **Name** ______________________

Activity A **Date** ____________ **Period** ____________

Match the following terms and identifying phrases.

G 1. A rod used to keep the blade sharp as you work.

D 2. Called a melon baller by home cooks.

B 3. A type of steel used to make knives that sharpens well but rusts easily. It also loses its shine and discolors quickly after its first use.

I 4. The portion of the knife blade that extends into the handle of the knife.

F 5. A type of steel used to make knives that is difficult to sharpen, but does not pit, rust, or discolor; and does not affect the flavor of foods.

E 6. Long-handled tool used to strain items or lift them out of liquid.

A 7. The thick metal collar on some knives that runs from the heel of the blade to the handle.

J 8. A flat, abrasive stone used to sharpen a knife once its edge is dull and worn.

C 9. A type of metal used to make most good quality professional knives.

H 10. A type of cutting board made from man-made material.

A. bolster
B. carbon steel
C. high-carbon stainless steel
D. Parisienne scoop
E. spider
F. stainless steel
G. steel
H. synthetic
I. tang
J. whetstone

The Art and Science of Knife Construction

Chapter 11 **Name** ______________________

Activity B **Date** __________ **Period** __________

Three types of metal—*carbon steel, stainless steel,* and *high-carbon stainless steel*—are used for knife blades. In the chart below, circle the metal(s) that best fits the description in the column on the left. Some answers include more than one metal.

Description of Metal	Type of Metal (circle all that apply)		
Does not rust or discolor.	carbon steel	**stainless steel**	**high-carbon stainless steel**
Easiest to sharpen to a finely honed edge.	**carbon steel**	stainless steel	high-carbon stainless steel
Loses its shine and discolors quickly after its first use.	**carbon steel**	stainless steel	high-carbon stainless steel
Metal of which most good quality professional knives are made.	carbon steel	stainless steel	**high-carbon stainless steel**
Can transfer a metallic flavor to foods.	**carbon steel**	stainless steel	high-carbon stainless steel
Is so hard, it is difficult to sharpen and keep sharp.	carbon steel	**stainless steel**	high-carbon stainless steel
Will rust if left in a damp place.	**carbon steel**	stainless steel	high-carbon stainless steel

Answer the following questions about knife construction.

1. What is a full tang? A full tang extends all the way to the end of the knife handle as one continuous piece of metal.

2. Why is a knife with a full tang better than one with a rattail tang? The blade with a rattail tang often becomes loose within the handle and the knife is not safe to use.

3. What is the specific purpose of a bolster? The bolster acts to strengthen the blade at a stress point where knife blades often crack or chip.

4. What is a balanced knife? A balanced knife is one in which the weight of the handle is balanced with the weight of the blade.

Reviewing Key Concepts

Chapter 11 **Name** ______________________________

Activity C **Date** ___________ **Period** ___________

Part 1: Using a Steel and Whetstone

Circle the clue in parentheses that best completes each of the following statements.

1. The steel (**is a rod used to keep the blade sharp as you work**) (**is a flat, abrasive stone used to sharpen a knife once its edge is dull and worn**).
2. When using a steel, use (**slight**) (**moderate**) (**full**) force when stroking the steel and keep the edge of the knife at a (**20**) (**45**) (**60**)-degree angle to the steel.
3. There are two methods for using a steel. In one method, you hold the steel in front of you and (**parallel**) (**perpendicular**) to your body. For the other method, place the tip of the steel on the cutting board and hold it so the steel is (**horizontal**) (**vertical**).
4. Both methods for using a steel require that the blade be honed (**only where worn**) (**the full length of the blade**).
5. The whetstone (**is a rod used to keep the blade sharp as you work**) (**is a flat, abrasive stone used to sharpen a knife once its edge is dull and worn**).
6. Most chefs lubricate the whetstone to make sharpening easier. Two lubricants typically used for sharpening in the professional kitchen are (**vegetable oil and butter**) (**olive oil and water**) (**mineral oil and water**).
7. When sharpening, begin with the (**fine**) (**coarse**) side of the stone.
8. When using the whetstone, hold the knife at a (**20**) (**45**) (**60**)-degree angle to the surface of the stone.
9. Begin with the heel of the blade in the (**lower right**) (**upper left**) corner of the stone. Repeat the process on the other side of the blade. Begin with the heel in the (**lower left**) (**upper right**) corner of the stone.
10. After using the stone, finish the edge by honing it on (**the fine side of the whetstone**) (**the coarse side of the whetstone**) (**the steel**).

(Continued)

Activity C *(Continued)* **Name** ______________________

Part 2: Knives in the Professional Kitchen

Match the following terms and identifying phrases.

__J__ 11. Has a long, narrow, flexible blade. Using a light sawing motion allows you to cut cooked meat and poultry into thin, even slices.

__K__ 12. Has an inwardly curved blade that makes the job of cutting vegetables into small football shapes easier.

__D__ 13. Is easily identified by its large rectangular blade, which is used for chopping.

__F__ 14. Have flexible blades, but are not sharp. Used for spreading coatings on food or as a spatula to turn food while cooking.

__L__ 15. A smaller version of the chef knife, typically with a blade between 5 and 7 inches long.

__B__ 16. Is the most used knife in any chef's knife kit and sometimes called a *French knife*. Has various length blades.

__A__ 17. Blade is about 6 inches long. Used for separating muscle from bone on meat or poultry, or for filleting and portioning fish.

__E__ 18. Not sharp, but has a pointed end, which is used to pry apart shells of oysters.

__G__ 19. Small, short-bladed knife designed to cut away skin or peel.

__C__ 20. Short knife with a 1-inch wide blade that tapers to an edge, but is not sharp. Used for opening clams, not for cutting.

__H__ 21. Also called a *butcher's knife*. Has a long, thick, highly curved blade.

__I__ 22. Has teeth like a saw and is used for cutting breads and pastries.

A. boning and filet knives
B. chef knife
C. clam knife
D. cleaver
E. oyster knife
F. palette knives and spreaders
G. paring knife
H. scimitar
I. serrated slice
J. slicer
K. tourné knife
L. utility knife

(Continued)

Activity C ***(Continued)*** **Name** ______________________________

Part 3: Hand Tools in the Professional Kitchen

Answer the following questions in the space provided.

23. Why have wooden cutting boards recently returned to commercial kitchens?

    Recent research shows hardwood cutting boards are less likely than synthetic boards to allow bacteria to grow.

24. For what type of task is the Parisienne scoop designed?

    Portioning foods into small ball shapes.

25. For what type of task can both a skimmer and a spider be used?

    To strain items or lift them out of liquid.

Part 4: Knife Storage and Safety

Answer the following questions in the space provided.

26. What are two goals of storing knives correctly?

    The goals are to protect the knives and keep cooks safe.

27. What are four things a chef or cook should do before storing a knife?

    The knife should be cleaned, rinsed, sanitized, and completely dry before storage.

28. How should knives be stored?

    Store knives in a knife holder that is sanitized regularly.

Notes

Knife Skills

12

Terminology

Chapter 12

Activity A

Name ______________________________

Date __________ **Period** __________

Match the following terms and identifying phrases.

Answer	Item		Term
I	1. A round slice cut from round food such as carrots. It is often ¼-inch (6 mm) thick.	A.	batonnet
A	2. Portion of food cut into stick shapes that are 2 x ¼ x ¼ inch (50 x 6 x 6 mm).	B.	brunoise
C	3. Portion of food cut into stick shapes that are 2 x ⅛ x ⅛ inch (50 x 3 x 3 mm).	C.	julienne
D	4. Portion of food cut first into sticks and then into cubes ¾ x ¾ x ¾ inch (2 x 2 x 2 cm).	D.	large dice
E	5. Portion of food cut first into sticks and then into cubes ½ x ½ x ½ inch (13 x 13 x 13 mm).	E.	medium dice
J	6. Portion of food cut first into sticks and then into cubes ¼ x ¼ x ¼ inch (6 x 6 x 6 mm).	F.	mincing
B	7. Portion of food cut first into sticks and then into cubes ⅛ x ⅛ x ⅛ inch (3 x 3 x 3 mm).	G.	paysanne
G	8. Portion of food cut first into sticks and then into rectangles ½ x ½ x ¼ inch (13 x 13 x 6 mm).	H.	proficient
F	9. The process of chopping food into very fine pieces.	I.	rondelle
K	10. A seven-sided football shape. Vegetables are often cut into this shape in high-end restaurants.	J.	small dice
H	11. Skilled at producing knife cuts.	K.	tourné

Numerical Patterns in Knife Cuts

Chapter 12 **Name** ____________________________

Activity B **Date** __________**Period**__________

Recognizing simple patterns in a numerical sequence or set of sequences can help you predict the next number or sequence. Some of the series of cuts used in the professional kitchen to prepare vegetables are examples of such sequences. Once you know the pattern, you can easily calculate the others.

One way to discover relationships in numerical sequences is to look for a pattern in the way each term relates to the one before it. For example, in the number sequence 0, 5, 10, 15, 20..., the pattern is that each term is 5 more than the one before it. It is reasonable to predict that the next number in the sequence would be 25.

A. Analyzing stick cut patterns

Analyze the patterns in the following two stick cuts, then answer the questions that follow.

Julienne: 2 x 1/8 x 1/8 inch

Batonnet: 2 x 1/4 x 1/4 inch

1. What stays the same in both cuts? **length**
   What changes? **size of sides**
2. What is the numerical difference between the size of the sides in the julienne and the batonnet? **Julienne is half the size of batonnet or 1/8 inch smaller.**
3. What is the pattern? **Each stick is the same length, but the sides are twice the size of the next smaller stick.**
4. Some chefs use a smaller variation of julienne that is 2 x 1/16 x 1/16 inch. If you add this cut to the sequence, does the pattern change? **No change.**

(Continued)

Activity B ***(Continued)*** **Name** ______________________

B. Analyzing dice cut patterns

Analyze the numerical pattern of the following dice cuts, then answer the questions that follow.

Brunoise: ⅛ x ⅛ x ⅛ inch

Small dice: ¼ x ¼ x ¼ inch

Medium dice: ½ x ½ x ½ inch

5. What is the pattern of the size of the dice cuts? Each dice is twice the size of the dice that comes before it.

6. The dimensions of large dice are ¾ x ¾ x ¾ inch. Does the large dice cut fit into the established pattern? Explain. No. The established pattern is that each dice is twice the size of the dice that comes before it. Twice the medium dice would be 1 x 1 x 1 inch, not ¾ x ¾ x ¾ inch.

7. What pattern can you describe to help you remember the dimensions of dice cuts? The three smallest dices follow the pattern of each being twice the size of the dice that comes before it. The large dice is the size of the small dice plus the medium dice or one-and-a-half times the size of the dice that comes before it.

Reviewing Key Concepts

Chapter 12 Name ____________________

Activity C Date __________ Period __________

Part 1: Preparing a Cutting Workstation

Circle the clue in parentheses that best completes each of the following statements.

1. Select a (**cleaned and dried**) (**cleaned and sanitized**) cutting board.
2. Place a (**damp**) (**dry**) towel between the cutting board and the (**vegetables**) (**worktable**).
3. Assess the height of the worktable and cutting board. If cutting board is too low, you can use a series of (**sheet trays**) (**towels**) to elevate it.
4. Select the appropriate knife and make sure the edge is (**sharp**) (**not too sharp**).
5. Stand facing the worktable. Feet should be (**shoulder-width apart**) (**close together**).

Part 2: Technique for Cutting with the Chef Knife

Read each statement below. Circle the letter *T* if the statement is true. If the statement is false, circle *F* and write the corrected statement on the lines that follow.

T F 6. Position the guiding hand on one or several smaller objects. Be sure the thumb and pinky are holding the objects securely and are behind the other fingers. The front fingers are curved.

____

____

T F 7. Place the flat side of the knife against the end joint of the front fingers of the guiding hand.

The flat side of the knife should be placed against the middle joint of the front fingers of the guiding hand.

T F 8. Gently glide the chef knife in the proper forward and backward motion until the tip of the blade is resting on the cutting board.

The proper motion is forward and down until the entire blade is resting on the cutting board.

T F 9. Lift the back end of the knife so that the tip remains pointing down. Slide the guiding hand back to the location of the next cut.

____

____

(Continued)

Activity C *(Continued)* **Name** ____________________

Part 3: Technique for Using the Boning Knife, Paring Knife, Slicer, and Serrated Bread Knife

Answer the following questions in the space provided.

10. Which of the following is *not* a correct technique for gripping a boning knife. B
    A. All the fingers grip the handle of the knife as if shaking someone's hand.
    B. The thumb and forefinger grasp the portion of the knife blade just next to the end of the handle.
    C. All the fingers except the index finger grip the handle. The index finger rests on the back of the blade.
    D. All the fingers wrap around the handle with the blade pointing down.
11. When using the chef's knife, the guiding hand directly guides the knife during cutting. When using a boning knife, what does the guiding hand do?
    Manipulates the fish or meat during the cutting process.
12. When making a tourné with a paring knife, do you draw the knife from top to bottom or bottom to top? top to bottom
13. Which is correct when making a tourné, making a series of even short cuts or one long continuous cut? one long continuous cut
14. After the first cut on the tourné, how much do you turn the vegetable before making the next cut? 1/7th revolution
15. How many equal sides should a finished tourné have? seven
16. The slicer and serrated bread knife are used in similar manners. The hand is wrapped around the handle like a handshake. How many fingers are kept on the blade?
    none
17. When using a slicer or serrated bread knife, should the knife stroke be a long and sawing motion or short with strong downward pressure?
    long and sawing motion
18. When using a slicer or serrated bread knife, should the knife hand be held tight or relaxed during slicing? relaxed

Notes

Smallwares

13

Terminology

Chapter 13 **Name** ______________________________

Activity A **Date** ____________ **Period** ____________

Circle the clue in parentheses that best completes each of the following statements.

1. A (**mandoline**) (**rondeau**) (**chinois**) is a wide pan with 6 to 8 inch (15 to 21 cm) sides and two looped handles.
2. A large bowl-shaped strainer used to drain large quantities of product is a (**mandoline**) (**rondeau**) (**colander**).
3. Sautoir is a sauté pan (**with sloped or rounded sides**) (**with straight sides**) (**also called a Griswold**).
4. Sauteuse is a sauté pan (**with sloped or rounded sides**) (**with straight sides**) (**also called a Griswold**).
5. A cone-shaped strainer used to remove lumps and particles from liquids such as sauces is a (**mandoline**) (**china cap**) (**rondeau**).
6. To cook foods gently in hot water, chefs use a (**china cap**) (**mandoline**) (**bain marie**).
7. Pots, pans, and other hand tools used to prepare food are called (**bain marie**) (**smallwares**) (**rondeau**).
8. (**Hotel pans**) (**Sheet pans**) (**Chinois**) are rectangular stainless steel pans used to hold food in steam tables, warmers, and refrigerators.
9. (**Hotel pans**) (**Sheet pans**) (**Chinois**) are larger, shallow pans used for baking and food storage.
10. A (**pot**) (**pan**) (**colander**) is a cooking container that is as tall, or taller, than it is wide.
11. A (**sautoir**) (**sauteuse**) (**chinois**) is a type of china cap that has a finely woven, metal mesh.
12. A (**pot**) (**pan**) (**chinois**) is a cooking container that is wider than it is tall.
13. To chop large quantities of food, chefs use a machine called a (**mandoline**) (**conduction**) (**buffalo chopper**).
14. A device used to slice food by pushing the food onto and across a sharp metal blade is a (**mandoline**) (**conduction**) (**buffalo chopper**).
15. (**Mandoline**) (**Conduction**) (**Bain marie**) is the term used to describe how well pots and pans transfer heat from the burner or oven to the food they contain.

Using a Scientific Approach to Evaluate Cookware

Chapter 13 Name ______________________________

Activity B Date ___________Period___________

Use your textbook as a resource to complete the charts below. Circle the term that best describes each property for that material. If the information is not available in your text, circle *Unknown*. When you have completed the charts, answer the questions that follow.

Copper				
Property	**Circle one for each property**			
Conduction	excellent	good	poor	unknown
Reacts with food	yes	no		unknown
Tarnish resistant	yes	no		unknown
Weight	heavy	medium	light	unknown
Cost	high	moderate	low	unknown

Aluminum				
Property	**Circle one for each property**			
Conduction	excellent	good	poor	unknown
Reacts with food	yes	no		unknown
Tarnish resistant	yes	no		unknown
Weight	heavy	medium	light	unknown
Cost	high	medium	low	unknown

Stainless Steel				
Property	**Circle one for each property**			
Conduction	excellent	good	poor	unknown
Reacts with food	yes	no		unknown
Tarnish resistant	yes	no		unknown
Weight	heavy	medium	light	unknown
Cost	high	medium	low	unknown

(Continued)

Activity B *(Continued)* **Name** ______________________

1. Aluminum is the most widely used material for commercial cookware. What factor(s) do you think contributes most to it being the preferred material? Explain your answer. Aluminum costs less than other materials and is lightweight.

2. Copper pans are often lined with stainless steel. What would be the advantage of that combination? The copper would conduct the heat well and the stainless steel lining would prevent the copper from reacting with the food.

3. The best stainless steel pans have copper bottoms. What would be the advantage of that combination? The stainless steel weighs less, is tarnish resistant, and doesn't react with food. The copper bottom will give the pan better heat conduction than a stainless steel bottom.

Reviewing Key Concepts

Chapter 13 **Name** ______________________________

Activity C **Date** ____________ **Period** ____________

Part 1: Measuring and Portioning Tasks

Circle the clue in parentheses that best completes each of the following statements.

1. Containers used for measuring volume come in several sizes. Their capacities range from one cup to several (**cups**) (**quarts**) (**gallons**).
2. Sets of measuring spoons are useful for measuring small amounts of ingredients such as (**sugar and salt**) (**herbs and spices**) (**sugar and spices**). Measuring spoons range in size from an eighth of a teaspoon up to (**one teaspoon**) (**one tablespoon**) (**two tablespoons**).
3. To measure large quantities of food when it is delivered to the kitchen, foodservice operations use a (**portion**) (**balance-beam**) (**receiving**) scale.
4. To measure small quantities and individual ingredients, foodservice operations use a (**portion**) (**balance-beam**) (**receiving**) scale.
5. A (**portion**) (**balance-beam**) (**receiving**) scale has two platforms and a set of counterweights.
6. Bakers and pastry chefs typically use a (**portion**) (**balance-beam**) (**receiving**) scale to measure large amounts of dry ingredients.
7. Some (**bimetallic coil**) (**laser**) (**thermocouple**) (**candy**) thermometers can be placed in an oven and the meter placed outside the oven so it can be easily monitored.
8. Another name for a deep-fat thermometer is the (**bimetallic coil**) (**laser**) (**thermocouple**) (**candy**) thermometer.
9. One disadvantage of the (**bimetallic coil**) (**laser**) (**thermocouple**) (**candy**) thermometer is that they only measure the temperature on the surface and not internally.

Part 2: Straining Equipment

Circle the clue in parentheses that best completes each of the following statements.

10. A (**china cap**) (**chinois**) is a type of (**china cap**) (**chinois**) that has a finely woven, metal mesh.
11. The sieve through which cooked foods, usually potatoes, are placed and forced through with the plunger is a (**drum sieve**) (**ricer**).

(Continued)

Activity C *(Continued)* **Name** ______________________

Part 3: Cutting and Processing Equipment

Match the following terms and identifying phrases.

__D__ 12. A hollow, metal box with different size teeth on each side. It's used for shredding vegetables, cheese, chocolate, citrus peel, and spices.

__F__ 13. A device used to slice food by pushing the food onto and across a sharp metal blade.

__A__ 14. A two-part machine consisting of a motorized base and a covered container. The food to be processed is placed in the container and a lid covers the top to prevent splash.

__G__ 15. An auger forces the food through a feed tube, past a rotating blade, and through the holes of the die. Used to process meat or other foods into various textures.

__E__ 16. A one-piece machine consisting of a motorized shaft with blades on the end. The shaft and the blades are immersed in a container of liquid to purée the product.

__B__ 17. Consists of a rotating bowl into which the food is placed. The bowl then passes under a set of rotating blades that chop the food into small pieces.

__H__ 18. Uses a rotating blade to slice foods thinly and evenly.

__C__ 19. Used primarily to grind, purée, and blend, but has cutting attachments that can produce shredded, julienned, and diced foods in a wide range of sizes.

A. bar blender
B. buffalo chopper
C. food processors
D. grater
E. immersion blender
F. mandoline
G. meat grinder
H. slicer

(Continued)

Activity C ***(Continued)*** **Name** ______________________

Part 4: Smallwares Storage and Kitchen Equipment Safety

Answer the following questions in the space provided.

20. What are four things a chef or cook should do before storing smallwares?

The smallwares should be cleaned, rinsed, sanitized, and completely dry before storage.

21. What are two ways smallwares are often stored?

They are hung up in the kitchen for easy access or stored in drawers or on shelves (invert if on shelves).

22. What is the OSHA regulation for usage of kitchen equipment for workers under 18 years of age?

People under 18 years of age are *not* **permitted to operate, clean, or repair power equipment such as meat slicers or bakery mixers.**

23. Name six things you should do before working with any dangerous equipment.

get trained on its proper use and safety, wear any personal protective equipment provided by the employer, use any machine guarding provided, ask for help if you are not sure how to do something, be aware that age restrictions exist for workers under the age of 18 for using or cleaning certain equipment, follow the manufacturer's instructions for machine use and cleaning

24. What should you do if a piece of kitchen equipment malfunctions?

Report any malfunctions—never try to fix machine jams or malfunctions yourself. Disconnect the power source and report the problem to your supervisor.

Large Equipment 14

Terminology

Chapter 14 **Name** ____________________

Activity A **Date** __________ **Period** __________

Match the following terms and identifying phrases.

H 1. The most common type of commercial cooktop. Pots or pans are placed on trivets directly over a gas flame burner.

L 2. A permanently fixed, large pot with double-walled construction. It is a quick and efficient way to heat large quantities of liquid because the interior is heated with pressurized steam.

E 3. A polished stainless steel cooktop on which food is cooked directly without pots or pans.

J 4. A list of tasks to be performed to ensure that equipment stays in proper working order.

A 5. A radiant heat source placed above the food to be cooked.

M 6. A device that responds to temperature changes and either turns the burner on or off.

K 7. Small broiler, less powerful than regular broilers, used only for browning food.

C 8. Oven with a fan that helps circulate the hot air inside the oven.

D 9. Range with a heavy cast-iron top that has a heat source located underneath the top. Pots and pans are placed on the top and heated by conduction.

B 10. Oven that uses heat and steam to cook foods.

F 11. Cooking appliance that has the radiant heat source located below the food and rack.

G 12. A cooktop that uses electromagnetic energy to heat special pots and pans.

I 13. To move back and forth very rapidly.

A. broiler
B. combination oven
C. convection oven
D. flattop range
E. griddle
F. grill
G. induction range
H. open-burner range
I. oscillate
J. preventive maintenance schedule
K. salamander
L. steam-jacketed kettle
M. thermostat

The Best Equipment for the Job

Chapter 14 **Name** ____________________

Activity B **Date** __________ **Period** __________

Select the appliance from the list that is best suited for each function described below. Write your answer in the space provided. Some terms will not be used.

broiler	griddle	salamander
combination oven	grill	steam-jacketed kettle
convection oven	open-burner range	tilt braiser
convection steamer	pressure fryer	
flattop range	pressure steamer	

Function	Cooking Appliance Recommended
1. Heats food in pots or pans while maintaining instant control of the heat.	open-burner range
2. Browns food rather than fully cooks it.	salamander
3. Quickly heats up to 100 gallons (379 L) of liquid.	steam-jacketed kettle
4. Uses several pots and pans at the same time; does not offer instant control of heat.	flattop range
5. Cooks food on a rack with heat source located below.	grill
6. Braises large quantities of product.	tilt braiser
7. Steams food that could be easily ruined by overcooking.	convection steamer
8. Roasts food, which is very vulnerable to drying out, as quickly as possible.	combination oven
9. Cooks eggs, sandwiches, and pancakes in a short-order establishment.	griddle
10. Cooks food on a rack with heat source located above.	broiler
11. Bakes foods at an even temperature.	convection oven

Reviewing Key Concepts

Chapter 14 **Name** ______________________

Activity C **Date** __________ **Period** __________

Part 1: Holding Equipment

Two common pieces of holding equipment are steam tables and warming cabinets. Place a check (✓) under the piece of equipment described in each statement.

Holding Equipment		
Description	**Steam Table**	**Warming Cabinet**
Is sometimes referred to by the French term *bain marie.*	✓	
May have features that maintain moisture in the cabinet.		✓
Is heated by an electric element.		✓
Holds hot food in hotel pans and metal inserts by surrounding them with hot water and steam.	✓	
May be heated by gas or electric.	✓	
Are placed in the area of the kitchen where food is plated for service.	✓	

Part 2: Fryers

Circle the clue in parentheses that best completes each of the following statements.

1. Deep fryers cook food by (**coating**) (**submerging**) (**basting**) them in hot fat.
2. Fryers are found in (**only fast-food**) (**only fine-dining**) (**most**) restaurants.
3. A fry kettle with a tightly sealed lid is called a (**deep fryer**) (**pressure fryer**) (**steam-jacketed kettle**).
4. Deep fryers are classified by the amount of (**chicken**) (**donuts**) (**fat**) they hold.
5. In a pressure fryer, the pressurized kettle fries food (**rapidly**) (**slowly**).

(Continued)

Activity C ***(Continued)*** **Name** ______________________

Part 3: Refrigeration

Identify the correct statement in each set of statements below. Place a check (✓) in the space before each correct statement.

6. __✓__ A. Refrigeration stores foods below 41°F (4°C).
   ______ B. Refrigeration stores foods at 0°F (-18°C).
   ______ C. Refrigeration stores foods above 32°F (0°C).

7. ______ A. Refrigerators are defined by their temperature range.
   __✓__ B. Refrigerators are defined by their size.
   ______ C. Refrigerators are defined by their shape.

8. ______ A. Freezers store foods below 41° F (4°C).
   __✓__ B. Freezers store foods at 0°F (-18°C).
   ______ C. Freezers store foods below 32°F (0°C).

9. __✓__ A. Refrigeration works by removing heat from the refrigerator compartment.
   ______ B. Refrigeration works by channeling cold air into the refrigerator compartment.

10. ______ A. Refrigeration equipment is typically located in one area in a commercial kitchen.
    __✓__ B. Refrigeration equipment is typically located throughout a commercial kitchen.

Part 4: Equipment Maintenance

Name three elements of a proper maintenance schedule for equipment found in commercial kitchens. Use your textbook as a resource.

11. (Answers can occur in any sequence.) A description of daily cleaning of the equipment

12. Weekly or monthly checks and adjustments such as lubrication of mechanisms and detailed cleaning

13. Monthly, quarterly, or annual service such as calibration of thermostats and maintenance of motors

15

Using Recipes

Terminology Crossword

Chapter 15 **Name** ____________________

Activity A **Date** ____________ **Period** ____________

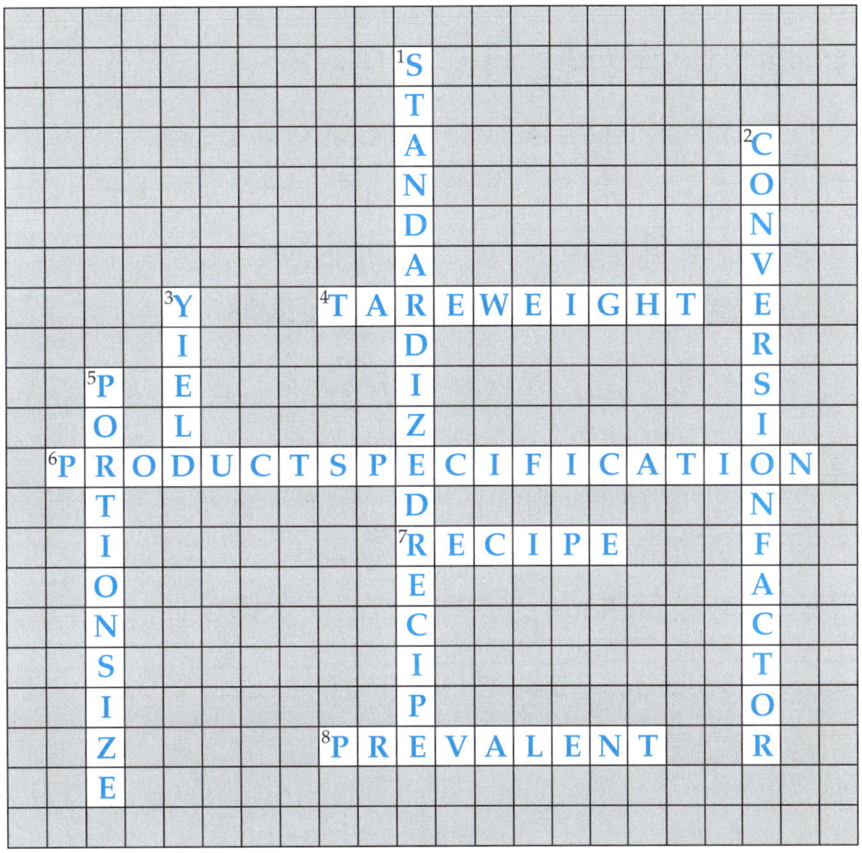

Across

4. Weight of the container that holds the ingredients being measured. (two words)
6. Detailed description of a product used in a foodservice operation. (two words)
7. A list of products and the amounts needed to prepare a dish followed by preparation instructions.
8. More widely accepted.

Down

1. Chefs and managers use this tool to create a dish that is uniform each time it is prepared. (two words)
2. A multiplier that adjusts the quantity of each ingredient in the original recipe to determine the quantities needed for the revised recipe. (two words)
3. Term used to describe the quantity or number of portions the recipe will produce.
5. Indicates the serving size that the chef expects to be served to each customer. (two words)

Changing Recipe Yield

Chapter 15 **Name** ____________________

Activity B **Date** __________ **Period** __________

To increase or decrease the yield of a recipe, you must accurately adjust the amounts of the ingredients listed in the original recipe. The first step is to determine the conversion factor. The second step is to multiply the amount of each ingredient in the original recipe by that factor.

Part 1: Determine Conversion Factors

Use the following formula to calculate conversion factors.

New Yield ÷ Old Yield = Conversion Factor

Write the equation and solve it to find the conversion factor for each situation below. Round answers two decimal places. (*Reminder: 5 or more rounds up.*)

1. Original recipe makes 12 portions; chef needs 32 portions.

   Equation: 32 ÷ 12 Conversion factor = 2.67

2. Original recipe makes 8 portions; chef needs 64 portions.

   Equation: 64 ÷ 8 Conversion factor = 8

3. Original recipe makes 40 portions; chef needs 10 portions.

   Equation: 10 ÷ 40 Conversion factor = 0.25

4. Original recipe makes 20 portions; chef needs 6 portions.

   Equation: 6 ÷ 20 Conversion factor = 0.30

5. Original recipe makes 18 portions; chef needs 126 portions.

   Equation: 126 ÷ 18 Conversion factor = 7

(Continued)

Activity B *(Continued)* **Name** ______________________

Part 2: Apply Conversion Factors

In the following problems, use the conversion factor to calculate the new quantity needed. Round off answers to two decimal places.

6. Conversion factor is 0.75 and the original quantity is 1 mL.

   New quantity needed = 0.75 mL

7. Conversion factor is 0.375 and the original quantity is 3 lb.

   New quantity needed = 1.13 lb.

8. Conversion factor is 4.5 and the original quantity is 6 oz.

   New quantity needed = 27 oz.

9. Conversion factor is 0.3 and the original quantity is 2.8 L.

   New quantity needed = 0.84 L

10. Conversion factor is 6 and the original quantity is 12 eggs.

    New quantity needed = 72 eggs

Part 3: Changing Yields

Calculate the following conversions to determine the ingredient amounts needed. Round answers to one decimal place.

11. The original soup recipe calls for 3.5 quarts of stock. The yield is 20 portions. How much stock will be needed to prepare 160 portions? 28 quarts

12. The original recipe calls for 7 pounds of veal. The yield is 12 portions. How much veal will be needed for 8 portions? 4.7 pounds

Reviewing Key Concepts

Chapter 15 **Name** ____________________

Activity C **Date** __________ **Period** __________

Part 1: Measurement and Units of Measure

Complete the list of terms below by writing the abbreviations for the units of measure in the parentheses. Then fill in the blanks in the statements that follow using the appropriate terms from the list. (Some terms will be used more than once, some will not be used at all.)

cup (c.)	liter (L)	pounds (lb.)
fluid ounce (fl. oz.)	milliliter (mL)	tablespoon (Tbsp.)
gram (g)	ounces (oz.)	volume
kilogram (kg)	pint (pt.)	weight

1. Two basic units of weight in the US system of measure are ___ounces___ and ___pounds___.
2. The basic unit of volume in the US system of measure is the ___fluid___ ___ounce___.
3. The basic unit of weight in the metric system of measure is the ___gram___.
4. The basic unit of volume in the metric system of measure is the ___liter___.
5. The two units of volume most often used in the metric system are the

   ___liter___ and ___milliliter___.
6. ___Weight___ is the preferred way to measure ingredients in the professional kitchen because it is more accurate and consistent than measuring by ___volume___.
7. Water and liquids that have a similar density to water, such as wine, stock, juice, and milk, can be measured using either volume or weight. In the US system, one fluid ounce of such liquids equals one ___ounce___ in weight. In the metric system, one milliliter of these liquids equals one ___gram___.

(Continued)

Activity C *(Continued)* **Name** ____________________

Part 2: Equivalents

Write the missing amounts and units in the spaces provided.

8. 1 fluid ounce = __30__ mL
9. 1 gallon = 3.8 __L__
10. 1 quart = 0.95 __L__
11. 1 tablespoon = __3__ teaspoons
12. 1 ounce = __28__ grams
13. 1 pound = __16__ ounces or 454 grams
14. 1 cup = __8__ fluid ounces
15. 1 gram = 0.035 __ounces__

Part 3: Standardized Recipes

Read each of the following statements and circle *S* if it describes a standardized recipe. Circle *H* if it is typical of a home recipe.

S (H) 16. Ingredients may not be listed separately from the preparation instructions.

(S) H 17. Ingredients are always separate from the preparation instructions.

S (H) 18. Number of portions may be given, but portion size is not described.

(S) H 19. Portion size is expressed in ounces, cups, or by count.

(S) H 20. Quantities of most products are measured by weight whenever possible.

S (H) 21. Quantities of most products are measured by volume.

(S) H 22. Provides detailed product descriptions including market form, size, grade, and brand.

S (H) 23. Provides only general, nonspecific names of products.

Part 4: Measuring Accurately

A. Measuring liquid and dry ingredients

Circle the clue in parentheses that best completes each of the following statements.

24. To measure dry ingredients by volume, (**overfill**) (**underfill**) the container and (**scrape off ingredients above the rim**) (**press down ingredients just below the rim**) (**gently shake the container to settle ingredients**).

25. To measure liquid ingredients, (**an opaque**) (**a clear**) container is best. Place the container on a level surface. To read the measurement, bend over so that the measuring line is (**at**) (**just above**) (**just below**) eye level.

(Continued)

Activity C ***(Continued)*** **Name** ______________________

B. Tare weight

Explain how to account for tare weight in each situation below.

26. You must measure out 1½ pounds of sugar. You have a metal bowl to hold the sugar, but the only scale available cannot be reset. How can you adjust for tare weight?

Weigh the empty bowl. Add the weight of the bowl to 1½ pounds to find what the total weight of the container and the sugar should be. Place the bowl on the scale and add sugar until the scale reads the desired total weight.

27. You want to measure a quantity of figs in a glass bowl. Your scale can be reset. What steps can you take to determine just the weight of the figs?

Place the empty bowl on the scale. Reset the weight indicator to read zero. Add the figs to the bowl until the desired weight of figs is reached.

C. Product specification

Answer the following questions in the space provided.

28. What is a product specification and why is it necessary?

A detailed description of a product used in foodservice. Product specification is necessary to ensure that the same size, quality, and type of product is used.

29. Name five typical product specifications for food products.

(Name five.) product, market form (fresh, frozen, dried, etc.), size, grade, brand

30. Suppose you are a restaurant chef and need to substitute one ingredient for another. What should you do first and why?

Consult your supervisor. Not all ingredient substitutions are easy. Some require other changes to the recipe. Others may introduce potential allergens that could be life-threatening to a customer.

Basic Preparations—Mise en Place

16

Terminology

Chapter 16 **Name** ______________________________

Activity A **Date** ___________ **Period** ___________

Match the following terms and identifying phrases. Terms may be used more than once.

Answer	Phrase	Terms
D	1. A vegetable-based seasoning made of two parts chopped onion, one part chopped carrot, and one part chopped celery.	A. chiffonade
A	2. Refers to thinly cut strips of leafy greens.	B. clarified butter
C	3. Refers to roughly dicing or chopping a product.	C. concassé
G	4. A variation of a vegetable-based seasoning made of three vegetables.	D. mirepoix
A	5. Certain leafy vegetables and fresh herbs can be cut into this.	E. mise en place
D	6. For even cooking, the three vegetables in this must be cut to the same size.	F. remedy
C	7. Is a technique for dicing tomatoes.	G. white mirepoix
G	8. Contains two parts chopped onion, one part chopped leek, and one part chopped celery.	
F	9. Correction of a recipe error during preparation.	
E	10. Refers to having all foods and equipment ready for a specific preparation before beginning it.	
B	11. Is ideal for higher temperature cooking.	
B	12. The fat portion of the butter, which has been separated from the water and milk solids.	
E	13. Can refer to a state of mental readiness.	

Calculating Butter to Clarified Butter Ratio

Chapter 16 | **Name** ______________________

Activity B | **Date** __________ **Period** __________

Clarified butter is one of the staples of professional kitchens. It is ideal for higher temperature cooking. To make clarified butter, you start with whole butter.

A. What makes up butter?

Butter has three basic parts—fat, water, and milk solids. Each part has distinctive properties. Clarified butter is the fat portion.

1. Create a key using a different pattern or color for each part to distinguish among the parts on the graph. In the blank below each key, write the percentage of the whole that each part makes up.

Key: Key: Key:

__80__% Fat __18__% Water __2__% Milk Solids

2. Complete the bar graph below to illustrate the percent each part represents.

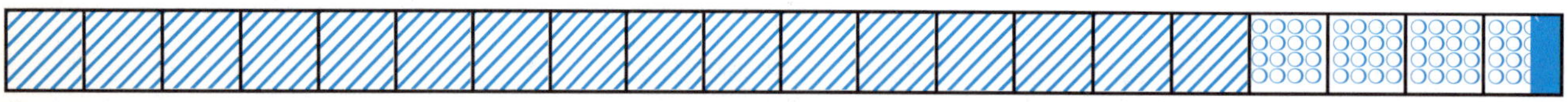

B. Calculating quantity of whole butter needed to achieve desired yield.

When butter is clarified, it yields about 75 percent clarified butter. You can use this percentage to calculate how much butter you would need to produce a given amount of clarified butter. For example, if you needed 12 ounces of clarified butter, you would ask the mathematical question: 12 is 75% of what number? Set up this question as an equation in which n represents the unknown quantity of butter needed to produce 12 ounces of clarified butter.

$\frac{12}{n} = \frac{75}{100}$ Cross multiply $\frac{12}{n} \times \frac{75}{100}$ $12 \times 100 = n \times 75$ $1200 = 75n$

Divide both sides by 75 to solve for n $\frac{1200}{75} = \frac{75n}{75}$ $1200 \div 75 = n$ $16 = n$

You would need to start with 16 ounces, or 1 pound, of butter to produce 12 ounces of clarified butter. Use this method to calculate how much butter to use to produce the amounts of clarified butter listed below. Show your calculations on a separate sheet of paper. Round answers to nearest whole number.

3. For 10 ounces of clarified butter, begin with ____13 ounces____ of butter.
4. For 18 ounces of clarified butter, begin with ____24 ounces____ of butter.
5. For 170 g of clarified butter, begin with ____227 grams____ of butter.

Reviewing Key Concepts

Chapter 16 **Name** ______________________

Activity C **Date** __________ **Period** __________

Part 1: Mise en Place

Place a check (✓) before each element below that is a part of mise en place.

__✓__ 1. Reviewing the menu or recipe and readying all food and equipment needed for a specific preparation before beginning it.

__✓__ 2. Setting up your station prior to service.

__✓__ 3. Chopping herbs and onions.

__✓__ 4. Getting your mind ready to work.

Part 2: Peeling, Mincing, Dicing, and Julienning Vegetables

Read each statement below. Circle the letter *T* if the statement is true. If the statement is false, circle *F* and write the corrected statement on the lines that follow.

T (F) 5. When peeling an onion, cut the onion horizontally halfway between root and stem.

When peeling an onion, cut the onion in half lengthwise through the root and stem.

(T) F 6. To remove the root of an onion, make a small triangular cut with tip of a knife.

____

(T) F 7. To dice onions, be sure the root end of the onion faces away from the knife.

____

T (F) 8. To peel a garlic clove, lay it on a cutting board, cover with the handle of a chef knife, and press firmly.

To peel a garlic clove, lay it on a cutting board, cover with the blade of a chef knife, and press firmly.

T (F) 9. The germ of garlic should be removed if it shows no sign of green.

The germ of garlic should be removed if it appears green.

(Continued)

Activity C *(Continued)* **Name** ______________________

(T) F 10. To mince garlic, begin by coarsely chopping the peeled cloves.

____

____

T (F) 11. To make garlic paste, sprinkle minced garlic with dash of sugar and press with the side of a knife blade. Repeatedly drag the knife across the garlic.

To make garlic paste, sprinkle minced garlic with dash of salt and press with the side of a knife blade. Repeatedly drag the knife across the garlic.

T (F) 12. For recipes that rely on a strong parsley flavor, wrung-out parsley works best.

For recipes that rely on a strong parsley flavor, wrung-out parsley is not recommended.

(T) F 13. To mince parsley, first wash and dry the parsley and then separate the parsley leaves from the stems.

____

____

T (F) 14. Parsley is wrung out before it is minced.

Parsley is wrung out after it is minced.

____

(T) F 15. Leeks are unique in that they are dirty on the inside as well as the outside.

____

____

T (F) 16. After trimming the root end of leeks, remove the dark green leaves all at once.

After trimming the root end of leeks, remove the dark green leaves one at a time.

____

(T) F 17. For leek halves or quarters, cut leeks in half lengthwise.

____

____

(Continued)

Activity C *(Continued)* **Name** ____________________

T (F) 18. To clean leeks, soak them in cold water for 10 to 15 minutes, then pour the leeks and soaking water into a colander to drain.

To clean leeks, soak them in cold water for 10 to 15 minutes, then scoop the leeks off the top of the water using a spider.

(T) F 19. To peel tomatoes, remove the core, cut an "X" through the skin of the opposite end, and plunge in boiling water for 30 seconds. Immediately place in ice water to cool.

(T) F 20. To seed tomatoes, first divide the tomato in half by cutting through the middle.

(T) F 21. Use the concassé technique for dicing tomatoes when you need roughly cut tomatoes.

(T) F 22. When preparing a fine dice tomato, the seeds remain inside as the flesh is trimmed off.

Part 3: Chiffonade Technique

Read each description below and write ***Yes*** in front of the accurate description and ***No*** in front of the inaccurate one.

no 23. To make a chiffonade, lay five to six leaves side by side on the cutting board. Cut across leaves with a sawing motion to make thin slices. Fluff the cuts to reveal the chiffonade.

yes 24. To make a chiffonade, lay five to six leaves in a stack on the cutting board. Tightly roll the stack. Cut thin slices across the roll. Unroll the cuts to reveal the chiffonade.

(Continued)

Activity C ***(Continued)*** **Name** ______________________________

Part 4: Clarified Butter

Letter the steps for clarifying butter below in sequential order. The first step should be labeled *A*. Some steps may not be used.

__D__ 25. Carefully pour the fat into a clean container.

__F__ 26. Ladle remaining fat from the water's surface.

__A__ 27. Place butter in metal container.

__B__ 28. Place the metal container in lightly simmering water.

______ 29. Stir after one minute.

__E__ 30. Stop pouring when the water becomes visible.

__C__ 31. When butter has melted, skim foam off the top using a ladle.

Kitchen Staples 17

Terminology

Chapter 17
Activity A

Name ______________________________

Date ____________ **Period** ____________

Match the following terms and identifying phrases.

Answer	Phrase
E	1. The green leafy parts of aromatic plants that are used to flavor foods.
L	2. The woody parts of plants, including seeds, bark, berries, buds, and roots that are used to flavor foods.
D	3. The flavorings or seasonings served with foods to enhance their flavor.
I	4. Foods that have been saturated with acid, usually vinegar, in order to preserve them.
J	5. Condiments made of a mixture of chopped or diced ingredients preserved in an acidic liquid.
C	6. A condiment made of preserved fruits and vegetables with an acidic, sweet and spicy flavor.
B	7. The bud of a bush that grows near the Mediterranean.
G	8. The fruit of the olive tree that is native to the Mediterranean region.
A	9. Small, oily ocean fish preserved by salting.
F	10. A liquid infused with different ingredients.
H	11. Spread throughout.
K	12. A combination of seasonings massaged into food to impart flavor.

A. anchovies
B. capers
C. chutney
D. condiment
E. herb
F. marinade
G. olives
H. permeate
I. pickle
J. relish
K. rub
L. spice

Reviewing Key Concepts

Chapter 17 **Name** ______________________

Activity B **Date** __________ **Period** __________

Part 1: Basic Seasonings

Match the following seasonings and identifying phrases. Some seasonings may be used more than once.

__B__ 1. Comes from chili peppers.

__C__ 2. Is used to season clear broths or consommés because it has no additives.

__D__ 3. Not used to season food, but baked shellfish is often served on a bed of it.

__F__ 4. Widely used in professional kitchens because it adds pepper flavor without black specks.

__A__ 5. The dried berrylike fruit of an Asian plant that is used whole, crushed, cracked, or ground.

__E__ 6. Is often referred to as granulated salt because it is in the form of fine granular crystals.

__B__ 7. Adds a very strong, hot, spicy flavor to dishes.

__C__ 8. Many chefs prefer to use it when sprinkling seasoning with their fingers.

A. black pepper
B. cayenne pepper
C. kosher salt
D. rock salt
E. table salt
F. white pepper

(Continued)

Activity B *(Continued)* **Name** ____________________

Part 2: Herbs

Match the following herbs and identifying phrases. Some herbs may be used more than once.

J 9. The classical garnish for fish and poultry.

F 10. Often used in pickling and is excellent with fish.

N 11. Essential for béarnaise sauce.

L, M 12. Goes well with poultry, pork, and game.

A, I 13. Used in tomato sauces.

B, O 14. Used to flavor stocks, soups, stews, and other savory dishes.

D 15. Has a delicate onion-garlic flavor.

E 16. Has a strong flavor with citrus tones and is commonly used in salsas.

K 17. Also called Italian parsley.

G 18. Has a flavor similar to a combination of thyme and oregano.

H 19. Garnish for desserts and used with lamb in Middle Eastern cuisines.

E 20. Its seeds are a spice called *coriander.*

L 21. Has stiff needles on a woody stem and a pinelike aroma.

I 22. Is popular in Italian, Greek, and Mexican cuisines and is actually wild marjoram.

C 23. Has delicate, lacy leaves with a light licorice flavor and is used in sauces.

A. basil
B. bay leaf
C. chervil
D. chives
E. cilantro
F. dill
G. marjoram
H. mint
I. oregano
J. parsley (curly)
K. parsley (flat-leaf)
L. rosemary
M. sage
N. tarragon
O. thyme

(Continued)

Activity B *(Continued)* **Name** ____________________

Part 3: Starches

Match the following starches and identifying phrases. Some starches may be used more than once.

A, B, C, E, F	24. Can be used as a thickening agent.	A. all-purpose flour
A, C, D, F	25. Can be used as a coating.	B. arrowroot
G	26. Is combined with all-purpose flour to make pasta.	C. bread crumbs
A	27. Appropriate for general purpose baking and cooking.	D. cornmeal
B	28. Looks identical to cornstarch.	E. cornstarch
F	29. Lends a light texture to sauces and coatings. Used for tempura batter.	F. rice flour
D	30. Milled from both yellow and white corn. Used for baking and coating.	G. semolina
C	31. Panko is a popular style of this starch.	

Part 4: Tomato Products

Rank the following tomato products from 1 to 5 in order of the concentration. The product with the greatest concentration should be "1."

4 tomato juice

1 tomato paste

3 tomato purée

5 fresh tomatoes

2 tomato sauce

Reviewing Key Concepts

Chapter 17 **Name** ______________________

Activity C **Date** __________ **Period** __________

Part 1: Spices

Match the following spices and identifying phrases. Some spices will not be used.

__D__ 1. The light green, pointed seeds of a plant grown in India that are used in curries, breads, and pastries.

__X__ 2. Star-shaped fruit of a tree grown in China that is important in Chinese cuisine.

__Y__ 3. Often used in rice dishes, curries, pickling, and prepared mustard, it is known for the bright yellow color it gives dishes.

__A__ 4. Also known as Jamaican pepper, it is often used in forcemeats, pickling, and baking.

__B__ 5. Has a strong licorice flavor and is commonly used in liquors and for baking.

__H__ 6. Dried, bark of a tropical tree with a sweet flavor that makes it popular for use in pastries and fruit dishes.

__W__ 7. Pale seeds of an annual plant native to India that are used in baked goods and vegetable dishes. The seeds are also ground to a paste to make tahini or pressed to extract oil.

__N__ 8. Greenish-brown seeds of a plant whose bulb is used as a vegetable. Seeds have a licorice flavor and are often used in sausages and pork dishes.

__Q__ 9. The red, veiny middle layer of the same seed that produces nutmeg with an intense spicy flavor. Used in desserts, baking, and some savory dishes.

__K__ 10. Seed of an annual plant that originated in the Middle East. Often used in chilies and curries, it is popular in Mexican, Indian, and Middle Eastern cookery.

__T__ 11. Powder ground from a variety of different red chile peppers.

__O__ 12. Root of a tropical plant that is used in powdered form for baking, but fresh in Asian cuisines.

__P__ 13. Berries of an evergreen tree that are used for game dishes and to flavor gin, marinades, and stews.

A. allspice
B. anise
C. caraway seeds
D. cardamom
E. cayenne pepper
F. celery seed
G. chile powder
H. cinnamon
I. cloves
J. coriander
K. cumin
L. curry powder
M. dill seed
N. fennel seed
O. ginger
P. juniper berries
Q. mace
R. mustard
S. nutmeg
T. paprika
U. poppy seeds
V. saffron
W. sesame seeds
X. star anise
Y. turmeric

(Continued)

Activity C *(Continued)* **Name** ____________________

Part 2: Sweeteners

Match the following sweeteners and identifying phrases.

F	14. Also known as sucrose, it is primarily used to add a sweet flavor to dishes.	A. brown sugar
B	15. Also known as glucose, its clear form has a neutral sweet flavor; the dark form is more robust.	B. corn syrup
D	16. Graded on color, clarity, and flavor with a light or amber color being most valued.	C. honey
A	17. Created by adding molasses back into refined sugar.	D. maple syrup
C	18. When substituted for sugar, gives the dish a distinctive flavor of the sweetener.	E. molasses
E	19. The liquid that is left over after refined sugar is extracted from sugarcane juice.	F. sugar

Part 3: Acid Ingredients and Condiments

Read each statement below. Circle the letter *T* if the statement is true. If the statement is false, circle *F* and write the corrected statement on the lines that follow.

(T) F 20. Vinegar can be made from any alcoholic beverage.

T (F) 21. Malt vinegar is often used as a condiment to baked foods in English cuisine.

Malt vinegar is often used as a condiment to fried foods in English cuisine.

T (F) 22. The acid content of bottled lemon juice and fresh lemon juice differ widely.

The acid content of bottled lemon juice and fresh lemon juice is relatively the same.

(T) F 23. Yellow, or salad style, mustard is a mild mixture. Its color comes from turmeric.

(Continued)

Activity C ***(Continued)*** **Name** ______________________

(T) F 24. The flavor of soy sauce is stronger, thicker, and more intense when the ratio of wheat to soybeans is high.

____

____

T (F) 25. Capers should not be rinsed before using them in a recipe.

Capers should be rinsed before using them in a recipe.

____

(T) F 26. Chutney is made of preserved fruits and vegetables. It has an acidic, sweet and spicy flavor.

____

____

T (F) 27. Olives are sometimes treated with sugar or vinegar to remove their bitter flavor.

Olives are sometimes treated with salt or lye to remove their bitter flavor.

____

(T) F 28. Green olives are picked underripe. Black olives are picked ripe.

____

____

T (F) 29. Anchovies are mostly sold as fillets canned in water.

Anchovies are mostly sold as fillets canned in oil.

____

(T) F 30. The flavor of Worcestershire sauce is derived from dozens of ingredients.

____

____

(T) F 31. Horseradish's strong burning flavor goes well with rich, fatty meats.

____

____

(Continued)

Activity C *(Continued)* **Name** ______________________

T (F) 32. All hot sauces are basically made from vinegar flavored with sweet peppers and salt.

All hot sauces are basically made from vinegar flavored with hot chile peppers and salt.

T (F) 33. The most common pickles used in American kitchens are kosher dill pickles, dill gherkins, and cornichons.

The most common pickles used in American kitchens are kosher dill pickles, sweet gherkins, and cornichons.

Part 4: Marinades and Dry Rubs

Answer the following questions in the space provided.

34. What is a marinade?

A marinade is a liquid that is infused with different ingredients in which foods are soaked in order to impart flavor before cooking.

35. How are marinades prepared?

Marinades are prepared in two ways: by simply mixing the ingredients together or cooking to combine the ingredients.

36. What types of ingredients are used in rubs and how do they season food?

Rubs are made from many different ingredients such as spices, herbs, salt, and sweeteners. They are applied to the outside of food and season only the exterior of the food.

Cooking Principles 18

Terminology

Chapter 18
Activity A

Name ____________________
Date __________ Period __________

Part 1

Match the following terms and identifying statements.

C 1. The browning that occurs when sugars are heated, resulting in a richer, more complex aroma and flavor.

G 2. A cooking method that uses a radiation from a heat source below the food.

I 3. Cooking food in a liquid at a relatively low temperature.

E 4. The process of preparing food for eating by applying heat.

K 5. A moist method that cooks a food product by surrounding it with steam vapor.

D 6. The manner in which heat energy travels through liquids and gases.

H 7. Cooking the food in enough hot fat to cover it half way.

A 8. Cooking food in liquid at its highest possible temperature.

J 9. Quickly cooking an item in a small amount of hot fat over high heat.

B 10. Cooking process that combines browning and simmering.

F 11. Process during which starches combine with hot liquid and absorb the liquid and swell.

A. boiling
B. braising
C. caramelization
D. convection
E. cooking
F. gelatinization
G. grilling
H. panfrying
I. poaching
J. sautéing
K. steaming

(Continued)

Activity A *(Continued)* **Name** ______________________________

Part 2

Match the following terms and identifying statements.

__E__ 12. To brown a food product. Often described by the French term *au gratin*.

__G__ 13. The method that cooks a food by surrounding it with hot air.

__I__ 14. Cooking food in a small amount of fat using low heat in order to soften the food without browning.

__D__ 15. A method that cooks food in enough hot fat to fully cover the item.

__H__ 16. Cooking food in liquid at a temperature just below boiling.

__B__ 17. Cooking by using a radiant heat source located above the food.

__C__ 18. The transfer of heat energy from one object to another through direct contact.

__A__ 19. The method used to cook foods in the oven with a certain amount of added moisture.

__F__ 20. The transfer of heat energy through waves.

A. baking
B. broiling
C. conduction
D. deep frying
E. gratiner
F. radiation
G. roasting
H. simmering
I. sweating

The Science of Cooking

Chapter 18 **Name** ______________________________

Activity B **Date** ___________ **Period** ___________

Part 1: The Chemistry of Cooking

Select the appropriate phrases from the following list to complete the chart below. Place the letter for each phrase in the appropriate box.

Chemical Changes Resulting from Cooking

A. Much of the connective tissue in meat becomes tender when it is properly cooked.

B. Heat causes sugars to caramelize.

C. Starches combine with hot liquid, and swell in a process called gelatinization.

D. The cell structure of most plants is broken down by heat.

E. When proteins are heated, they coagulate.

F. Amino acids, which make up proteins, change when heated, creating new flavors.

G. Most bacteria, fungi, and molds are killed at normal cooking temperatures.

H. Applying heat blends the flavors of multiple ingredients.

Cooking Chemistry	
Reasons for Cooking Foods	**Chemical Changes Resulting from Cooking**
Cooked food is safer to eat.	G
Cooked food is more digestible.	A, D
Cooking improves texture, taste, aroma, and appearance of food.	B, C, E, F, H

Identify what can happen when foods are cooked to excessive temperatures or for too long by completing the following statements on the lines provided.

1. When food is overcooked, nutrients are ______lost______.

2. When food is overcooked, sugars burn causing foods to taste ______bitter______.

3. When food is overcooked, moisture is lost and foods become ______dry______.

4. When food is overcooked, proteins can ______toughen______ or ______curdle______.

5. When food is overcooked, texture is destroyed and foods become either ______mushy and disintegrate______ or ______tough and stringy______.

6. When food is overcooked, the color of green vegetables ______is lost and turns brown______.

(Continued)

Activity B *(Continued)* **Name** ______________________

Part 2: The Physics of Cooking

Circle the clue in parentheses that best completes each of the following statements.

7. The transfer of heat energy through waves is referred to as (**conduction**) (**convection**) (**radiation**).
8. The transfer of heat energy from one object to another through direct contact is referred to as (**conduction**) (**convection**) (**radiation**).
9. The transfer of heat energy through liquids and gases is referred to as (**conduction**) (**convection**) (**radiation**).
10. The flames of a broiler transferring heat to food being cooked is an example of heat transfer by (**conduction**) (**convection**) (**radiation**).
11. A pot of boiling liquid being stirred is an example of heat transfer by (**conduction**) (**convection**) (**radiation**).
12. Microwaves also cook food by (**conduction**) (**convection**) (**radiation**).
13. Food cooking in a pan on a range is an example of heat transfer by (**conduction**) (**convection**) (**radiation**).
14. The natural rising of warm air to the top of an oven and the descending of the cooler air to the bottom of the oven is an example of heat transfer by (**conduction**) (**convection**) (**radiation**).

Cooking Methods

Chapter 18 **Name** ______________________________

Activity C **Date** ____________ **Period** ____________

For each cooking example given in the chart, select the appropriate cooking method from the list below and write it in the middle column. In the last column, circle the correct classification—**dry heat method (DHM), moist heat method (MHM), combination method (CM)**—for that cooking method.

Cooking Methods

baking	deep frying	poaching	simmering
boiling	grilling	roasting	steaming
braising	panfrying	sautéing	stewing
broiling			

Cooking Methods

Cooking Example	Cooking Method	Classification *(Circle one)*
Food is browned on all sides in fat, then liquid is added and food is simmered.	braising	(DHM) (MHM) **(CM)**
Food is quickly cooked in a small amount of hot fat over high heat.	sautéing	**(DHM)** (MHM) (CM)
Food is cooked in enough hot fat to fully cover the food item.	deep frying	**(DHM)** (MHM) (CM)
Food is cooked by surrounding it with steam vapor.	steaming	(DHM) **(MHM)** (CM)
Food is cooked in enough hot fat to cover the food item halfway.	panfrying	**(DHM)** (MHM) (CM)
Food is cut in small pieces and cooked in enough liquid for them to float freely during the process.	stewing	(DHM) (MHM) **(CM)**
Some moisture is added to food and then it is cooked in the oven.	baking	**(DHM)** (MHM) (CM)
Food is cooked by surrounding it with hot air.	roasting	**(DHM)** (MHM) (CM)
Food to be cooked is placed on a pan or a grill and then placed under the heat source.	broiling	**(DHM)** (MHM) (CM)
Food is cooked over a heat source.	grilling	**(DHM)** (MHM) (CM)
Food is cooked in liquid at a temperature just below boiling.	simmering	(DHM) **(MHM)** (CM)
Food is cooked in a liquid at a relatively low temperature.	poaching	(DHM) **(MHM)** (CM)
Food is cooked in liquid at its highest possible temperature.	boiling	(DHM) **(MHM)** (CM)

Notes

19

Salads and Dressings

Terminology

Chapter 19 **Name** ______________________

Activity A **Date** __________ **Period** __________

Match the following terms and identifying phrases. Some terms may be used more than once.

B 1. Usually made up of four parts—base, body, dressing, and garnish.

A 2. When cooked items are mixed with mayonnaise.

I 3. A salad of greens and various raw vegetables such as cucumbers, carrots, and tomatoes.

J 4. A mixture of three parts oil to one part vinegar.

E 5. A cold sauce that is an emulsion of oil and vinegar stabilized with egg yolk and mustard.

B 6. Also known as a plated salad.

I 7. May be served with any kind of dressing, which can be either tossed with the salad or served on the side.

D 8. Cooked foods mixed with a vinaigrette.

F 9. A mixture of baby lettuces.

C 10. A mixture of two liquids that don't naturally mix, such as oil and vinegar.

E 11. Important in the cold kitchen because it is often used as a base for dressings or cold sauces.

C 12. Made up of tiny droplets of one ingredient suspended in another ingredient.

G 13. The roof of the mouth.

H 14. Heating food at a temperature for a period of time that distroys unsafe organisms.

A. bound salad
B. composed salad
C. emulsion
D. marinated salad
E. mayonnaise
F. mesclun
G. palate
H. pasturize
I. simple salad
J. vinaigrette

Identifying Salads and Their Ingredients

Chapter 19 **Name** ______________________________

Activity B **Date** ____________**Period**____________

Part 1: Types of Salads on the Menu

Circle the clue in parentheses that best completes each of the following statements.

1. The traditional purpose salads have served on the menu is as (**an entrée**) (**an appetizer**) (**a dessert**).
2. Green salad paired with portions of cooked chicken, seafood, or meat is an example of (**an appetizer salad**) (**a main course salad**) (**a bar salad**).
3. Restaurant operators like salad bars because ingredient costs are relatively (**high**) (**low**) and labor costs are (**increased**) (**decreased**).
4. When salad ingredients are assembled in a particular arrangement, the finished salad is a (**simple salad**) (**composed salad**) (**bound salad**) (**marinated salad**).
5. A salad of greens and various raw vegetables such as cucumbers, carrots, and tomatoes is a (**simple salad**) (**composed salad**) (**bound salad**) (**marinated salad**).
6. A plated salad is also called a (**simple salad**) (**composed salad**) (**bound salad**) (**marinated salad**).
7. When cooked items are mixed with mayonnaise, they are referred to as (**simple salad**) (**composed salad**) (**bound salad**) (**marinated salad**).
8. Regardless of the ingredients, a (**simple salad**) (**composed salad**) (**bound salad**) (**marinated salad**) usually includes the following four parts: base, body, dressing, garnish.
9. When cooked foods are mixed with a vinaigrette, they are commonly called a (**simple salad**) (**composed salad**) (**bound salad**) (**marinated salad**).
10. Tossing simple salads with dressing too (**forcefully**) (**far in advance**) (**gently**) will cause the salad greens to wilt.

(Continued)

Activity B *(Continued)* **Name** ______________________

Part 2: Salad Greens

Match the following salad greens with the identifying phrases.

C	11. Soft green leaves form a loose head with creamy-colored inner leaves. The leaves have a delicate texture and cupped shape.	A. Belgian endive
A	12. Tightly packed, elongated head of white leaves with yellow tips and a bitter flavor.	B. bibb lettuce
I	13. Red lettuce with white stems and veins, and a bitter flavor.	C. Boston lettuce
M	14. Tender little shoots of various plants such as alfalfa, mung beans, radishes, and mustard.	D. curly endive
G	15. Large, tender, ruffled bunches of bright green leaves with a mild flavor. Used in salads, sandwiches, and for lining plates and platters.	E. escarole
B	16. Developed in Kentucky, this lettuce has color and texture similar to Boston lettuce but forms a smaller head. One whole head is often served as a single portion.	F. iceberg lettuce
F	17. With crisp leaves and round shape, this is the most popular variety of lettuce in the United States.	G. leaf lettuce
E	18. This loosely formed head of flat, curly edged leaves that are dark green at the tip and yellowish white at the base is often prepared as a hot vegetable in Italian cuisine.	H. mesclun
K	19. With an elongated, tightly packed head with round-tipped leaves and crisp ribs, it is the second most popular lettuce in the United States.	I. radicchio
H	20. A mixture of baby lettuces that is often purchased cut, washed, mixed, and ready to use.	J. red leaf lettuce
L	21. Can be purchased in bunches or cello pack. Fibrous stems should be removed and leaves washed several times, however, the smaller, tender leaves are best for salads.	K. romaine lettuce
J	22. Has the same texture and flavor as green leaf lettuce but with reddish-brown color at the tip of the leaves.	L. spinach
N	23. The classic plate garnish for red meats, but also used in salads. Has a peppery flavor.	M. sprouts
D	24. Crisp ribs create narrow leaves with a curly edge. Outer leaves are deep green with a pale yellow core. It has a bitter flavor and is usually served as part of a mix.	N. watercress

Purchase and Preparation

Chapter 19 **Name** ____________________

Activity C **Date** __________ **Period** __________

Part 1: Buying Lettuce

Circle the clue in parentheses that best completes each of the following statements.

1. Compared to other produce, lettuce is (**more**) (**less**) subject to fluctuations in quality and price.
2. Produce wholesalers generally sell lettuce by (**weight**) (**head**).
3. The waste from trimming or damaged leaves (**affects**) (**does not affect**) cost.
4. The lowest priced lettuce is (**always**) (**never**) (**not always**) the best buy.
5. The cost of ready-to-eat greens is (**lower**) (**higher**) than traditional greens.
6. Using ready-to-eat greens results in (**more prep time but less waste**) (**less prep time but more waste**) (**less prep time and less waste**).

Part 2: Preparing Salad Greens

Read each statement below. Circle the letter *T* if the statement is true. If the statement is false, circle *F* and write the corrected statement on the lines that follow.

T F 7. In a commercial kitchen, lettuce and greens are washed under running water.

Lettuce and greens are best washed by submersion, not under running water.

____

T F 8. The cores on head lettuce and the thick stems on leafy greens should be removed.

____

____

T F 9. The best method for drying greens is to pat them with absorbent paper towel.

The best option for drying greens is to spin them dry with a salad spinner.

____

(Continued)

Activity C ***(Continued)*** **Name** ____________________

T (F) 10. Because cutting lettuce with most knives causes oxidation, lettuce should always be torn, never cut.

Most chefs use knives that would not cause oxidation and cutting lettuce with a knife is more efficient than tearing it by hand.

(T) F 11. Wilted, outer leaves should be removed and discarded.

T (F) 12. In most cases, lettuce leaves should be kept whole for salads.

Lettuce should be cut into bite-size pieces.

Part 3: Dressings and Salad Preparation

Circle the clue in parentheses that best completes each of the following statements.

13. In vinaigrette, the task of the acidic vinegar is to (**enhance**) (**cut**) (**dissolve**) the fat, add another taste sensation, and (**help**) (**stop**) the oil from coating the palate.
14. The secret to preparing a good vinaigrette is balance between fat, acid, and other seasonings. The best ratio is usually (**two parts vinegar to one part oil**) (**one part oil to one part vinegar**) (**three parts oil to one part vinegar**) by volume.
15. It is important to stir simple vinaigrette (**well**) (**immediately**) before servings.
16. An emulsion is a mixture of two liquids that (**do not naturally**) (**naturally and easily**) mix.
17. Adding egg or egg yolk to mayonnaise (**separates**) (**stabilizes**) oil and vinegar.
18. The standard proportion for making mayonnaise is (**one-half**) (**one**) (**one and one-half**) egg yolk to (**one-half**) (**one**) (**one and one-half**) cup of oil.
19. The consistency of most emulsified dressings is (**thicker than**) (**thinner than**) (**about the same as**) mayonnaise.
20. The ingredient that makes up the biggest percent of most salad dressings is (**vinegar**) (**oil**) (**spices**).
21. The source of a particular oil, vinegar, or mustard (**can**) (**cannot**) noticeably alter the flavor of a salad dressing.

(Continued)

Activity C ***(Continued)*** **Name** ______________________

22. Mustard helps to (**separate**) (**cut**) (**emulsify**) mayonnaise and other emulsified dressings.
23. One yolk is roughly equivalent to (**one fluid ounce**) (**one tablespoon**) of pasteurized egg products, which are commonly used in commercial kitchens.
24. Keeping salad ingredients (**chilled**) (**at room temperature**) helps keep them sanitary.
25. (**Warm**) (**Chill**) salad plates before plating to avoid (**wilting**) (**frosting**) greens.
26. Use gloves or utensils to handle salad ingredients because it is (**unstable**) (**ready-to-eat**) food.
27. Mix tossed salads with dressing (**as close to service as possible**) (**as early as possible before service**).
28. When applying salad dressings, the rule is use just enough to (**cover the bottom of the bowl**) (**lightly coat the greens**).

Fruit Identification

20

Terminology

Chapter 20 **Name** ______________________

Activity A **Date** __________ **Period** __________

Match the following terms and identifying phrases.

Part 1

H	1. The weight of the packaging alone.	A.	bushel
J	2. Same grade as *Choice* for canned or frozen fruits.	B.	case
A	3. A volume measuring 35.24 liters or about 2200 cubic inches.	C.	count
D	4. The total weight of a container and the product.	D.	gross weight
E	5. A large bulk-packed case.	E.	lug
B	6. A box or container of varying size. May be made of cardboard, wood, plastic, or foam.	F.	net weight
G	7. Equivalent to one-fourth bushel.	G.	peck
I	8. Same grade as *Fancy* for canned or frozen fruits.	H.	tare weight
C	9. A specific number of pieces of uniform-sized produce in a case or container.	I.	US Grade A
F	10. The weight of the product without the packaging.	J.	US Grade B

(Continued)

Activity A *(Continued)* **Name** ____________________

Part 2

Match the following terms and identifying phrases.

B 11. A shallow single-layered case used for delicate products such as berries and figs.

A 12. A wooden case.

G 13. Same grade as *Standard* for canned or frozen fruits.

C 14. Evaluating a food against a uniform set of quality standards.

F 15. The federal agency that imposes standards for the quality and safety of food products in the United States.

D 16. The offspring of two different plant varieties.

E 17. Fruit or fruit pieces that are flash frozen before packing to retain their original shape.

A. crate
B. flat
C. grading
D. hybrid
E. individually quick frozen
F. USDA
G. US Grade C

Identifying Quality Fruits

Chapter 20 Name ______________________

Activity B Date __________ Period __________

Part 1: Identifying Fruits

Circle the clue in parentheses that best completes each of the following statements.

1. Oranges named for the navel-like protrusion near their stem are (**Valencia**) (**navel**) (**blood**).
2. The most important variety of orange is (**Valencia**) (**navel**) (**blood**).
3. Citrus fruits named for the deep red color of their flesh are (**tangerines**) (**blood oranges**).
4. Grapefruit fall into one of two categories based on (**flavor**) (**the color of their flesh**).
5. The most popular variety of apple in the United States is (**Fuji**) (**Gala**) (**Red Delicious**).
6. (**Braeburn**) (**Golden Delicious**) (**Cortland**) is *not* an all purpose apple.
7. Northern Spy, Spartan, and Granny Smith are (**cooking**) (**eating**) (**all purpose**) apples.
8. (**Seckel**) (**Asian**) (**Anjou**) are sweet, firm, crisp, and fragrant round shaped pears.
9. Cherries are classified into two main categories: (**light and dark**) (**sweet and sour**).
10. (**Bing**) (**Rainier**) (**Montmorency**) cherries are noted for bright red skin and juicy fruit.
11. The classification of peaches is based on (**color**) (**how difficult it is to remove their pits**).
12. A nectarine is a (**fuzzless peach**) (**type of stone fruit**) (**cross of a peach and a plum**).
13. Berries are some of the (**cheapest**) (**most expensive**) fruits in the commercial kitchen.
14. Tiny red seedless grapes that form in long clusters are (**Ribier**) (**Corinth**) (**Concord**) grapes.
15. The three melons commonly used in the commercial kitchen are (**Crenshaw, casaba, and cantaloupe**) (**honeydew, watermelon, and cantaloupe**) (**watermelon, casaba, and cantaloupe**).
16. The (**Cavendish**) (**plantain**) (**finger**) banana is the most common variety eaten in the United States.
17. Calimyrna, Mission, and Kadota are the most popular variety of (**kiwifruit**) (**figs**) (**dates**).
18. A small reddish-skinned fruit that has a white inner flesh with sweet, juicy, subtle flavor; originally grown in China is the (**kumquat**) (**lychee**) (**Kiwano**).
19. An oval fruit that looks like a five point star when sliced is (**carambola**) (**cherimoya**).
20. A small thumb-sized citrus fruit with almost no juice is (**kumquat**) (**lychee**) (**kiwano**).

(Continued)

Activity B ***(Continued)*** **Name** ______________________________

Part 2: Quality Factors for Selection

Circle the clue in parentheses that best completes each of the following statements.

21. **(Heavier)** **(Lighter)** citrus fruit generally has greater juice content.
22. **(Smooth)** **(Bumpy)** -skinned oranges are easier to peel and best for eating out of hand.
23. **(Smooth)** **(Bumpy)** -skinned oranges are hard to peel and reserved for juicing.
24. Green spots on grapefruit skin **(are)** **(are not)** a sign that the fruit is unripe.
25. When buying lemons look for **(fine-textured)** **(rough-textured)** skin and relatively **(light)** **(heavy)** weight for their size.
26. In lemons, **(deep)** **(light)** yellow color is a sign of maturity and **(less)** **(more)** acid.
27. Select apples that feel **(soft)** **(firm)** to the touch and have color appropriate for the variety.
28. For cooking, baking, and applesauce choose **(sweet, soft fleshed)** **(firm, tart)** apples.
29. For eating choose **(sweet, soft-fleshed)** **(firm, tart)** apples.
30. Ripe pears should **(resist slightly)** **(yield slightly)** to a gentle squeeze.
31. Many chefs prefer to buy pears **(fully ripened on the tree)** **(immature to ripen themselves)**.
32. When choosing apricots, choose fruit that is **(green)** **(yellow)** and **(hard)** **(slightly soft)**.
33. Quality peaches **(should)** **(should not)** have a fragrant aroma.
34. The deep red on orange color of nectarines **(is)** **(is not)** a sign of ripeness.
35. Plums should have good color for their variety and **(resist)** **(yield)** slightly to pressure.
36. Berries should be **(soft)** **(firm)** and **(bright)** **(even)** colored.
37. Juice stains at the bottom of the berry container are a sign that the berries are **(ripe)** **(deteriorating)**.
38. Select cranberries with bright red color and a **(hard)** **(soft)** **(springy)** texture.
39. Select **(compact)** **(loose)** bunches of grapes with **(moist, pliable)** **(dry, brittle)** stems.
40. Ripeness in cantaloupe **(can)** **(cannot)** be determined by its fragrance.
41. Regardless of the color of the outer rind, the best sign of watermelon ripeness is a pale **(green)** **(yellow)** underside.
42. Ripe papayas have skin that is at least half **(yellow)** **(red)**.
43. The only sure way to determine pineapple ripeness is to **(squeeze)** **(taste)** them.
44. Persimmons are rather **(soft)** **(firm)** when ripe.
45. Fragrance **(is)** **(is not)** a sign of ripeness in persimmons.

Fresh in Season or Processed?

Chapter 20 **Name** ______________________________

Activity C **Date** ___________ **Period** ___________

Part 1: Seasons for Fresh Fruits

Next to each month in the chart below, write the letters of every fruit that is in season during that period.

A. apricots
B. Bartlett pears
C. blackberries
D. blood oranges
E. blueberries
F. cherries
G. Cortland apples
H. cranberries
I. currents
J. figs
K. Gala apples
L. Granny Smith apples
M. honeydew melons
N. lemons
O. McIntosh apples
P. navel oranges
Q. papaya
R. peaches
S. pineapples
T. plums
U. raspberries
V. Rome Beauty apples
W. strawberries
X. Valencia oranges

Month	Fruits in Season
January	H, K, L, N, O, P, Q, S, V
February	K, L, N, O, P, Q, S, V, X
March	D, K, L, N, O, P, Q, S, V, X
April	D, L, N, O, P, Q, S, V, X
May	D, J, L, M, N, O, P, Q, R, S, T, U, V, W, X
June	A, C, E, F, I, J, L, M, N, O, Q, R, S, T, U, V, W, X
July	A, B, C, E, F, I, J, L, M, N, Q, R, S, T, U, V, W, X
August	B, C, E, F, I, J, K, L, M, N, Q, R, S, T, U, X
September	B, C, E, G, H, J, K, L, M, N, O, Q, R, S, T, V, X
October	B, G, H, J, K, L, M, N, O, Q, R, S, T, V, X
November	B, G, H, K, L, M, N, O, P, Q, S, V
December	B, H, K, L, N, O, P, Q, S, V

(Continued)

Activity C *(Continued)* **Name** ______________________

Part 2: Drying Fruits

Circle the clue in parentheses that best completes each of the following statements.

1. Raisins are dried **(grapes)** **(green grapes)** **(plums)** **(currents)**.
2. Prunes are dried **(grapes)** **(green grapes)** **(plums)** **(currents)**.
3. Sultanas are dried **(grapes)** **(green grapes)** **(plums)** **(currents)**.
4. Some dried fruits are treated with **(carbon dioxide)** **(sulfur dioxide)** to preserve their color and stop spoilage.
5. Keep dried fruits in **(an open)** **(a sealed)** container to preserve their flavor.
6. Many dried fruits are rehydrated or **(warmed)** **(moistened)** before using.

Part 3: Canned Fruits

Circle the clue in parentheses that best completes each of the following statements.

7. The flavor of canned fruits is usually consistent all year long because the fruits are usually packed at the **(beginning)** **(peak)** **(end)** of the season.
8. Fruit packed in **(water)** **(syrup)** retains more of the natural flavors of the fruit.
9. Fruit packed in **(water)** **(syrup)** is less likely to be broken or crushed.
10. The canning process preserves foods from spoilage until the can is opened and **(the fruit begins to dry)** **(the vacuum is broken)**.

Part 4: Frozen Fruits

Circle the clue in parentheses that best completes each of the following statements.

11. Frozen fruits retain **(more)** **(less)** flavor of fresh fruit than dry fruit retains.
12. Individually quick frozen (IQF) fruits are flash frozen **(before)** **(after)** packing and they tend to **(lose)** **(retain)** their original shape.
13. Adding sugar adds flavor and keeps fruit **(fully frozen)** **(from fully freezing)**.

Fruit Preparation

21

Terminology

Chapter 21

Activity A

Name ______________________

Date __________ **Period** __________

Match the following terms and identifying phrases. Then, circle the clue in parentheses that best completes the description.

C 1. A decoration added to a dish to make it (**sanitary**) (**attractive**).

E 2. The white, spongy inner part of (**citrus**) (**acidulating**) fruits.

B 3. Briefly cooking an item in (**simmering**) (**boiling**) water.

A 4. The process of (**adding acid to**) (**removing acid from**) an item.

F 5. To reconstitute or return some of the liquid removed from the fruit in the (**cooking**) (**preparation**) (**drying**) process.

D 6. The browning of (**all**) (**certain**) fruits once they are cut and exposed to the air.

H 7. The colorful, outermost part of the skin of (**citrus**) (**acidulating**) fruits.

G 8. An individual segment of any citrus fruit (**with**) (**without**) skin, pith, seeds, or membrane.

A. acidulation
B. blanching
C. garnish
D. oxidation
E. pith
F. plumping
G. suprême
H. zest

Preparing Fruit

Chapter 21 **Name** ______________________

Activity B **Date** __________ **Period** __________

Match each fruit group to the preparation technique that is most appropriate.

A. apples and pears
B. apples, pears, bananas, avocados
C. apples, pears, mangoes, and papayas
D. berries
E. cherries
F. citrus fruits
G. melons
H. melons, pineapples, citrus fruits, and kiwis
I. peaches, nectarines, and plums
J. peaches and nectarines
K. pineapples

1. K

Peeling and Coring

- Cut off the top and bottom.
- Trim the skin following the contour of the fruit from top to bottom.
- Continue working around the fruit until the skin is removed.
- Shave enough skin to remove the eyes.
- Cut the fruit in quarters lengthwise.
- Cut away from the fibrous core.

2. A

Coring

- Using a knife, cut the fruit in quarters through the stem.
- Cut out the core and seeds with a knife.
- Continue to cut into smaller pieces if desired.

3. D

Washing

- Gently submerge in cold water.
- Drain.
- Wash as close to time of service as possible to avoid fruit getting mushy.

4. F

Zesting

- Use a special tool called a zester to remove the outermost part of the fruit skin in fine julienne strips.
- If a zester is not available, use a peeler or a grater to remove the outermost part of the skin.

5. B

Acidulating

- Dip or brush cut fruit with one tablespoon of lemon juice to one quart of water.
- Dip rather then soak the fruit.

(Continued)

Activity B *(Continued)* **Name** ______________________

6. J

Removing Skin by Blanching
• Drop into rapidly boiling water for a few moments. • Place in cold water to cool down.

7. H

Removing Skin with Knife
• Use utility knife or flexible boning knife to remove skin. • Cut as little of the flesh as possible. Fruits should retain their rounded shape.

8. G

Peeling and Seeding
• Using a flexible knife, cut off the top and bottom. • With a slicing motion, trim the skin following the rounded contour of the fruit from top to bottom. • Continue trimming around the fruit until all the skin and rind is removed. • Cut the peeled fruit in half and scrape out the seeds with a spoon.

9. C

Removing Skin with a Peeler
• Use a stationary or swivel peeler to remove skin.

10. I

Pitting
• Use a paring knife and cut through the skin and flesh to the pit. • Cut to the pit a full 360 degrees. • Gently twist the two halves of the fruit in opposite directions until they separate. • Use the tip of a paring knife to remove the pit from the fruit.

11. E

Pitting
• Using the special tool designed for the purpose, push the pit through the flesh. • The fruit should remain uncrushed.

Fruit Presentation and Cooking

Chapter 21 **Name** ____________________

Activity C **Date** __________ **Period** __________

Part 1: Preparing Fruit Garnishes

Circle the clue in parentheses that best completes each of the following statements.

A. Parisiennes and citrus slices

1. The tool used to make Parisiennes is sometimes called a (**melon baller**) (**melon scoop**). Press the Parisienne scoop (**just into the surface of**) (**well into**) the fruit before turning it to make a perfectly round sphere, making sure to place one scoop close to the next to (**protect the shape**) (**minimize waste**).

2. Citrus slices can be made more interesting by cutting channels (**parallel**) (**perpendicular**) to the direction the slices will be cut. This exposes alternating stripes of white (**pith**) (**flesh**) and colorful (**flesh**) (**zest**) once the fruit is cut into thin slices.

3. Citrus slices can be turned into twists by cutting the slice from center to the outer edge and bending the halves in the (**same**) (**opposite**) direction.

B. Fruit crowns

4. Grip a paring knife on the blade at a point that is about the length of the (**diameter**) (**radius**) of the piece of fruit.

5. Hold the knife at a 45°angle to an imaginary line around the (**top**) (**middle**) (**bottom**) of the fruit. Insert the tip of the knife and push in until it reaches the center.

6. Hold the knife at (**a similar**) (**an opposing**) 45° angle and make a cut adjacent to the first one. Make sure the cuts (**overlap**) (**do not overlap**) slightly.

7. Continue these zigzag cuts around the fruit until you reach the starting point. Each cut (**should slightly**) (**should never**) intersect its adjacent cuts. Pull halves apart.

C. Fruit fans

8. To make a fruit fan, cut a (**flat**) (**rounded**) side on the bottom of a piece of fruit for stability. Make a slice at a (**45°**) (**90°**) angle to the cutting board. Cut through all but a small portion of the fruit.

9. Make additional slices (**parallel**) (**perpendicular**) to the first slice making sure to leave each slice (**partially attached**) (**totally attached**) to a small portion.

10. Press on the piece of fruit in the (**opposite**) (**same**) direction as the slices to open the fan.

(Continued)

Activity C ***(Continued)*** **Name** ______________________

Part 2: Cooking Fruit

Read each statement below. Circle the letter *T* if the statement is true. If the statement is false, circle *F* and write the corrected statement on the lines that follow.

T (F) 11. Fruits can be poached, steamed, or fried, but should never be baked, grilled, or sautéed.

Fruits can be cooked using any method.

T (F) 12. The cooking process preserves the fruit's rigid cell structure.

Cooking breaks down the fruit's rigid cell structure to make it tender.

(T) F 13. The degree of ripeness affects cooking time.

T (F) 14. In general, cooked fruits should still be firm when pierced with a fork or tip of a knife.

They should be tender.

(T) F 15. Dried fruits are plumped to return some of the liquid removed from the fruit in the drying process.

T (F) 16. Plumping is done by soaking the dried fruit in cold liquid or simmering them in liquid.

Plumping is done by soaking them in *hot* liquid or simmering.

Notes

Cold Sandwiches 22

Terminology

Chapter 22 Name ____________________

Activity A Date __________ Period __________

Circle the clue in parentheses that best completes each of the following statements.

1. (**À la Carte**) (**Baguette**) (**Pullman loaf**) is bread that is finely textured and cuts into square slices.
2. A preparation that involves a number of ingredients placed on, in, or between bread is referred to as a (**canapé**) (**Pullman loaf**) (**sandwich**).
3. The most common rolled sandwich today is the (**à la carte**) (**canapé**) (**wrap**).
4. A system in which food is prepared only when an order is received from the service staff is referred to as preparing food (**à la carte**) (**Danish sandwich**) (**baguette**).
5. Various ingredients rolled in a tortilla are called a (**canapé**) (**finger sandwich**) (**wrap**).
6. A category of sandwiches that includes tea sandwiches is (**à la carte**) (**finger sandwiches**) (**canapé**).
7. (**À la carte**) (**Danish sandwich**) (**Canapé**) sandwich stations are designed with speed in mind.
8. (**Baguette**) (**Pullman loaf**) (**Finger sandwich**) is the name for a long, thin French bread.
9. Neat, open-faced sandwiches that often include strongly flavored foods are referred to as (**Danish sandwiches**) (**finger sandwiches**) (**tea sandwiches**).
10. Small, bite-size, well-garnished, and attractive hors d'oeuvres that come in many different forms are referred to as (**à la carte**) (**canapés**) (**finger sandwiches**).
11. (**Canapé**) (**Danish sandwiches**) (**Tea sandwiches**) are small, closed-faced sandwiches made with crustless bread and trimmed to neat shapes.
12. A (**baguette**) (**Pullman loaf**) (**wrap**) is baked inside a mold with a cover.

Sandwich Types and Attributes

Chapter 22 **Name** ____________________

Activity B **Date** __________ **Period** __________

Part 1: Types of Sandwiches

List the five types of sandwiches in alphabetical order on the lines lettered A through E. Then, match the sandwich types with the identifying phrases.

E 1. After soft white bread has been flattened with a rolling pin, ingredients are then rolled tightly in the flattened bread.

C 2. A single slice of a small-diameter loaf of rye bread is spread with cream cheese and neatly topped with smoked salmon.

A 3. A bite-sized round of bread buttered and topped with a thin slice of cucumber.

B 4. A club sandwich.

D 5. A single slice of whole-grain bread is topped with lettuce and thin slices of avocado then sprinkled with lemon juice.

A. canapés

B closed

C. finger

D. open faced

E. rolled

Part 2: Attributes of Sandwiches

Chapter 22 names five attributes of successful and delicious sandwiches. Complete the following chart with the name of the attribute that corresponds to each of the chef's sandwich-making choices.

Chef's Sandwich Making Choices	Sandwich Attribute Achieved
6. Carefully spread the bread thinly with mayonnaise and lightly drizzle top of sandwich ingredients with olive oil.	moisture
7. Lightly sprinkle the top layer of ingredients with finely minced ripe tomatoes and green pepper.	appearance
8. Placed ingredients neatly and precisely on the bread making sure that the ingredients would not fall out when the sandwich was held.	easy to eat
9. Selected strongly flavored condiments and ripe vegetables to add to the sandwich ingredients.	flavor
10. Topped soft cheese with thin slices of crisp radish.	texture

Sandwich Ingredients and Assembly

Chapter 22 **Name** ____________________

Activity C **Date** __________ **Period** __________

Part 1: Sandwich Ingredients

Read each statement below. Circle the letter *T* if the statement is true. If the statement is false, circle *F* and write the corrected statement on the lines that follow.

(T) F 1. All sandwiches include some type of bread.

____

____

T (F) 2. Type of bread is always a choice regardless of the type of sandwich.

Certain sandwiches require specific breads.

____

T (F) 3. Sturdy, country-style loaves are ideal for delicate sandwiches like tea sandwiches.

Tender breads are ideal for delicate tea sandwiches.

____

T (F) 4. Originally served as breakfast rolls in France, focaccia are light crescent-shaped rolls that are often used for sandwiches today.

Croissants are light crescent-shaped rolls.

____

(T) F 5. Spreads prevent wet fillings from soaking into the bread because they are high in fat.

____

____

(T) F 6. Bound salad sandwiches do not need a spread.

____

____

T (F) 7. Sandwiches are usually named after the bread rather than the filling.

Sandwiches are usually named after the filling.

____

Activity C *(Continued)* **Name** ______________________

T (F) 8. Many sandwich fillings are high carbohydrate ingredients, which means sanitation practices must be rigorously followed when preparing sandwiches.

Many sandwich fillings are high protein ingredients.

(T) F 9. Cheeses can add moisture as well as flavor and texture to a sandwich.

T (F) 10. Garnishes need to look good, but flavor is usually not important.

It is important to choose a garnish that complements the flavor of the sandwich ingredients.

Part 2: Sandwich Assembly

A. Sandwich assembly strategies

Circle the clue in parentheses that best completes each of the following statements.

11. À la carte assembly strategies are also called (**self-serve**) (**made to order**).
12. In an à la carte assembly, all sandwich ingredients should be (**nearby**) (**within easy reach**).
13. À la carte sandwich stations should have a consistent (**alternating**) (**linear**) workflow.
14. In an à la carte sandwich station, the cutting board should be (**compact so as to not take up too much room**) (**large enough to hold several sandwiches at a time**).
15. Preportioned ingredients (**have no place**) (**save valuable time**) in an à la carte sandwich station.
16. Sandwich bars constitute a type of buffet because (**customers serve themselves**) (**customers selections are made to order**).
17. Sneeze guards are mandated by law for (**aesthetic**) (**health**) reasons.
18. Sandwich bars have become increasingly popular (**dinner**) (**lunch**) options.
19. Sandwich bars should be (**kept stocked**) (**replenished only during peak times**).

(Continued)

Activity C *(Continued)* **Name** ______________________________

B. Sandwich assembly line

In the spaces provided, briefly describe what tasks each cook in a five-station assembly line might perform to prepare a closed sandwich with mayonnaise, lettuce, cheese, cucumbers, minced olives, and mustard. The finished sandwich is wrapped in plastic and boxed.

Assembly Line Workers	Sandwich Assembly Tasks
20. First cook	**(Answers may vary.) Spreads mayonnaise on one slice of bread.**
21. Second cook	**(Answers may vary.) Places lettuce on mayonnaise and tops with cheese.**
22. Third cook	**(Answers may vary.) Adds a layer of cucumber slices on top of cheese.**
23. Fourth cook	**(Answers may vary.) Sprinkles minced olives on cucumbers and spreads mustard on second slice of bread and places on sandwich.**
24. Fifth cook	**(Answers may vary.) Wraps and boxes sandwich.**

Notes

Stocks

23

Crossword

Chapter 23

Activity A

Name ______________________________

Date ___________**Period**___________

Across

1. A concentrated instant powder or paste that dissolves in hot water to make a stocklike liquid.
2. One of two names for stocklike preparations that are made with a larger proportion of meat than bone and a greater variety of vegetables.
3. An animal protein that when dissolved in a hot liquid adds to a rich mouthfeel.
6. A bundle of fresh herbs tied to a piece of celery, leek, or carrot. (two words)
9. Dissolving the browned bits off the bottom of pan when preparing brown stock.
10. A highly flavored liquid made by simmering bones with vegetables, herbs, and spices.

Down

1. Stock made from roasted bones and roasted or sautéed mirepoix. (two words)
4. The process of placing bones in cold water, bringing the water to a boil, and then discarding water.
5. Stocks made using poultry, fish, or veal bones. (two words)
6. One of two names for stocklike preparations that are made with a larger proportion of meat than bone and a greater variety of vegetables.
7. French name for fish stock.
8. A small cheesecloth bag containing herbs and spices.

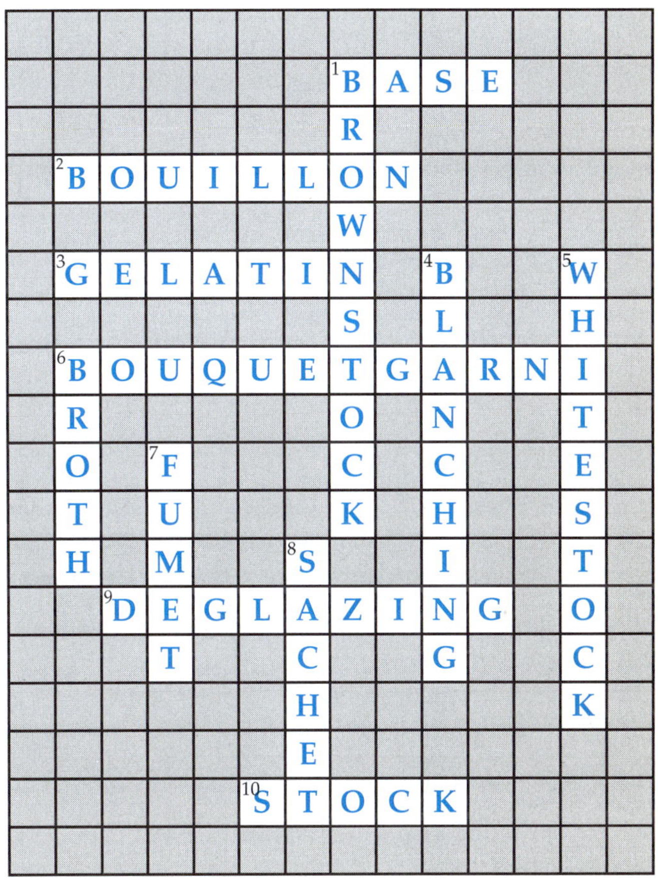

1 BASE
2 BOUILLON
3 GELATIN
6 BOUQUETGARNI
9 DEGLAZING
10 STOCK
1 BROWNSTOCK
4 BLANCHING
5 WHITESTOCK
6 BROTH
7 FUMET
8 SACHET

The Chemistry of Collagen

Chapter 23 Name ____________________

Activity B Date __________ Period__________

Extracting collagen from bones is an essential step in making full-bodied stock. Place a check (✓) next to the best choice in each step below.

Step 1. To produce a full-bodied beef stock, you should use bones from animals with the highest collagen levels. Which of the bones described will yield the highest levels of collagen?	
_____ Bones from mature animals.	__✓__ Bones from young animals.

↓

Step 2. Certain parts of animals have higher levels of collagen than others. Which parts of the animal will yield the most collagen for your beef stock?	
__✓__ Joints and feet	_____ Ribs and leg bones

↓

Step 3. Bones are simmered in liquid to create stock. Which choice of liquids will best brighten the stock's flavor and improve its clarity?	
_____ Water only.	__✓__ Water and small amount of wine.

↓

Step 4. For bones to supply the best flavor to the stock, the right amount of liquid must be used. How much liquid should be used to extract the best flavor when simmering bones for stock?	
_____ Enough liquid to cover the bones halfway.	__✓__ Enough liquid to cover bones with one to two inches of liquid.

↓

Step 5. Gelatin is a protein that is derived from collagen and gives stock mouthfeel. How long should bones be simmered to extract sufficient gelatin to produce a beef stock?	
__✓__ Bring stock to a boil and then simmer for at least 10 hours.	_____ Bring stock to a boil and then simmer for 3 to 5 hours.

↓

Step 6. After collagen turns into gelatin in your stock, what happens to it?	
__✓__ The gelatin dissolves into the simmering liquid.	______ The gelatin rises to the surface and needs to be skimmed off.

Reviewing Key Concepts

Chapter 23 **Name** ____________________

Activity C **Date** __________ **Period** __________

Part 1: Stock Ingredients and Attributes

Circle the clue in parentheses that best completes each of the following statements.

1. Nutritive ingredients of stock are (**meat and bones**) (**bones and water**) (**bones and gelatin**).
2. Meats add (**mouthfeel**) (**flavor**) (**body**) to stock, while bones add (**mouthfeel**) (**flavor**) (**body**).
3. Aromatic ingredients of stock include (**salt, spices, and herbs**) (**vegetables, salt, and herbs**) (**vegetables, herbs, and spices**). To improve and strengthen flavor of stocks, they are (**heated to a rapid boil to reduce**) (**simmered a greater length of time**).
4. The universal vegetable flavoring in stock is mirepoix, which is a (**specific combination of vegetables**) (**paste made of boiled down vegetables**) (**combination of mushrooms and tomatoes**).
5. Most stocks are flavored with three herbs (**bay leaf, rosemary, and sage**) (**thyme, bay leaf, and parsley**) (**rosemary, parsley, and thyme**).
6. The nutritive and aromatic ingredients of stock are typically simmered in water. Sometimes wine is added, which (**brightens the flavor, but clouds the stock**) (**adds acidity that brightens the stock's flavor and improves overall clarity**) (**cuts acidity, which clears the stock**).
7. All well made stocks share the following four attributes: (**body, spices, color, and lightness**) (**flavor, color, taste, and body**) (**color, clarity, flavor, and body**).
8. Vegetable stocks are not true stocks because they are (**not flavorful**) (**used only for vegetarian cuisine**) (**not made from bones**).
9. The difference between white and brown vegetable stock is that in white vegetable stock vegetables are first raw or (**baked**) (**panfried**) (**sautéed**), and in brown vegetable stock vegetables are first (**boiled**) (**browned**) (**sautéed**).
10. Vegetable stocks differ from meat-based stocks in one important way—(**they have less flavor**) (**they are more acidic**) (**they contain no gelatin**).
11. Vegetable stocks lack the (**mouthfeel**) (**flavor**) (**clarity**) of meat-based stocks.

Activity C *(Continued)* **Name** ______________________

Part 2: Bouillons, Broths, Bases, and Stocks

Read each statement below. Circle the letter *T* if the statement is true. If the statement is false, circle *F* and write the corrected statement on the lines that follow.

(T) F 12. One ingredient that is not added to stock is salt.

T (F) 13. White stocks are made using poultry, fish, or beef.

White stocks are made using poultry, fish, or veal.

(T) F 14. Bones are the principal, or most important nutritive ingredient in stock.

T (F) 15. Gelatin is the animal protein that when dissolved in a hot liquid adds a rich flavor to stock.

When dissolved in hot liquid, gelatin adds a rich *mouthfeel.*

(T) F 16. Deglazing greatly improves the flavor and color of a stock.

T (F) 17. Bouillons and broths are prepared using different preparation processes.

Bouillons and broths are two names for the same process.

T (F) 18. Bouillons and broths have a bone-to-meat ratio that is greater than that of stocks.

Bouillons and broths have a meat-to-bone ratio that is greater than that of stocks.

(Continued)

Activity C ***(Continued)*** **Name** ______________________

T (F) 19. Bouillons and broths typically require a more limited use of vegetables.

A greater variety of vegetables can be used for bouillons and broths.

(T) F 20. Broths and bouillons are classically reserved for soup production.

T (F) 21. The process for making broths and bouillons is specifically different from the process for making stocks.

Both brown and white bouillons and broths can be prepared using a procedure that mirrors the basic stock procedure.

(T) F 22. A base is a concentrated instant powder or paste that dissolves in hot water to make a stock-like liquid.

T (F) 23. Bases are slightly more expensive than stocks made from scratch.

Many bases are less expensive than stocks made from scratch.

(T) F 24. Most bases are limited in their use in sauce making because they contain salt.

T (F) 25. Bases that list fat as their first ingredient tend to be the highest quality.

Bases that require refrigeration after opening and list meat or meat juices as their first ingredient tend to be the highest quality.

Notes

Sauces

24

Terminology

Chapter 24 **Name** ____________________

Activity A **Date** __________ **Period** __________

Part 1

Match the following terms and identifying phrases.

__G__ 1. A yolk and cream mixture that is used to thicken liquids.

__B__ 2. When this happens to egg or milk mixtures, the liquid and solid portions separate from each other.

__J__ 3. A slurry made with flour.

__A__ 4. A thickening sauce made from puréed fruits or vegetables.

__H__ 5. Thickened liquids that complement other foods.

__I__ 6. A method of gradually warming the temperature of egg yolks before adding them to a hot sauce.

__E__ 7. A hot emulsified sauce that combines egg yolks and warm clarified butter.

__F__ 8. A reduced brown stock that is thickened with cornstarch or arrowroot slurry.

__D__ 9. A sauce that is made from a mother sauce.

__C__ 10. Is classically made by reducing espagnole sauce to proper nappé consistency.

A. coulis
B. curdle
C. demi-glace sauce
D. derivative sauce
E. hollandaise sauce
F. jus lié
G. liaison
H. sauce
I. tempering
J. whitewash

(Continued)

Activity A *(Continued)* **Name** ____________________

Part 2

Match the following terms and identifying phrases.

F 11. The consistency of a sauce when it is thick enough to coat the back of a spoon.

I 12. A mixture of cold liquid and starch used to thicken sauces.

E 13. In the French sauce system, each of the five base sauces from which other sauces are produced.

H 14. A mixture of equal parts flour and fat by weight that is cooked to varying degrees of doneness and used to thicken liquids.

A 15. Classic name for white sauce.

G 16. A small onion that is speared with several whole cloves pushed through a bay leaf.

C 17. Made by slowly reducing brown stock, a small amount of tomato product, mirepoix, and brown roux for hours.

J 18. A sauce that is made by thickening a white stock with a blond roux.

B 19. A mixture of softened whole butter and flour.

D 20. Uniform throughout.

A. béchamel sauce
B. beurre manié
C. espagnole sauce
D. homogenous
E. mother sauce
F. nappé
G. onion piqué
H. roux
I. slurry
J. velouté sauce

Roux Ratios

Chapter 24 **Name** ____________________________

Activity B **Date** ____________ **Period** ____________

Ratios describe the relationship between two or more numbers. Chefs use ratios when thickening sauces. For example, when using roux to thicken liquid into a sauce, the amount of roux to liquid can be expressed as a ratio. For the very lightest sauces, chefs use 8 ounces of roux for every 1 gallon (128 oz.) of liquid. This ratio is written 8 to 128. This ratio can also be written 8:128 or 8/128. (*Remember, the backslash in a fraction or ratio is the same as saying "divide by."*)

But what if you only need to thicken 32 ounces of liquid? How would you calculate how much roux you need to make a light sauce? Start by calculating how much roux is needed per one ounce of liquid. You know that to make a light sauce you need

8 oz. roux per 128 oz. liquid

This can be written as a ratio

$$\frac{8}{128}$$

The ratio can be written as a division problem

$$\text{8 oz. roux} \div \text{128 oz. liquid} = \frac{\text{0.0625 oz. roux}}{\text{oz. liquid}}$$

Now you can calculate how much roux the chef needs to thicken 32 ounces of liquid to light consistency. If you know how much roux is needed per ounce of liquid, you simply multiply the ounces of liquid by that amount

$$\frac{\text{0.0625 oz. roux}}{\cancel{\text{oz. liquid}}} \times 32\ \cancel{\text{oz. liquid}} = \text{2 oz. roux}$$

1. **A medium sauce recipe calls for 1 gallon of liquid thickened with 12 ounces of roux. Answer the following questions about the roux ratio for this preparation.**

   What is the ratio of roux to liquid? 12:128

   How much roux is needed to thicken one ounce of liquid to a medium sauce consistency? 12 oz. roux ÷ 128 oz. liquid = 0.09375 oz. roux/oz. liquid

   Calculate how much roux is needed to thicken 96 ounces of liquid to medium sauce consistency. 96 oz. liquid x 0.09375 oz. roux/oz. liquid = 9 oz. roux

(Continued)

Activity B ***(Continued)*** **Name** ______________________

2. A thick sauce recipe calls for 1 gallon of liquid thickened with 20 ounces of roux. Answer the following questions about the roux ratio for this preparation.

What is the ratio of roux to liquid? 20:128

How much roux is needed to thicken one ounce of liquid to a thick sauce consistency?

20 oz. roux ÷ 128 oz. liquid = 0.15625 oz. roux/oz. liquid

Calculate how much roux is needed to thicken 48 ounces of liquid to thick sauce consistency.

48 oz. liquid x 0.15625 oz. roux/oz. liquid = 7.5 oz. roux

Reviewing Key Concepts

Chapter 24 Name ____________________

Activity C Date __________ Period __________

Part 1: The Five Roles of Sauces

Circle the clue in parentheses that best completes each of the following statements.

1. Two elements that sauces add, which improve the appearance of food are (**color and liquidness**) (**color and shine**) (**color and milkiness**).
2. (**Visual appeal**) (**Olfactory appeal**) (**Texture appeal**) is an element that sauces can add to a simple center of a plate item that allows the dish to command a higher value on the menu.
3. Sauces add richness to food especially sauces that are high in (**jus lié**) (**nappé**) (**fat**).
4. Sauces contribute flavors that (**disguise**) (**reduce**) (**complement**) or accent the flavors of a particular dish.
5. Sauces add (**texture**) (**moisture**) (**body**) to keep the dish from tasting dry and unappetizing.

Part 2: Thickening Agents

Match the following terms and identifying phrases.

H 6. Thickens liquids very quickly, but if liquid is not stirred as it is added, lumps may form.

E 7. This agent thickens by adding finely ground fruits, vegetables, seeds, or nuts.

D 8. This method requires egg yolk, mustard, or natural emulsifiers to hold it together.

C 9. This thickening agent is often mixed with a small amount of cream and must be added to the sauce gradually or curdling may result.

G 10. The three types of this thickener are all made from the same proportions of fat and flour.

A 11. Can be used to thicken sauces at the last minute, but can produce a flavor of raw flour.

B 12. Rarely used method today because it produces a somewhat pasty texture.

F 13. This method concentrates flavor as well as thickens liquid.

A. beurre manié
B. bread
C. egg yolk
D. emulsion
E. purée
F. reduction
G. roux
H. slurry

(Continued)

Activity C *(Continued)* **Name** ______________________

Part 3: Classic System of Mother and Derivative Sauces

Use terms from the list to complete the chart that follows.

Allemande sauce	Cheddar sauce	White sauce
Béarnaise sauce	Fresh herbs sauce	White stock
Bordelaise sauce	Hollandaise sauce	
Brown stock	Tomato sauce	

Classical French Sauce System		
Mother Sauce	**Key Ingredient(s)**	**Derivative Sauces**
I. Brown sauce	A. **Brown stock**	1. **Bordelaise sauce** 2. Robert sauce
II. **Hollandaise sauce**	A. Egg yolks B. Clarified butter	1. **Béarnaise sauce** 2. Chantilly sauce
III. **Tomato sauce**	A. Tomatoes B. Flavoring agents such as herbs	1. Paprika and cream sauce 2. **Fresh herbs sauce**
IV. Velouté sauce	A. **White stock** B. Blond roux	1. **Allemande sauce** 2. Suprême sauce
V. **White sauce**	A. White roux B. Onion C. Bay leaf D. Nutmeg	1. **Cheddar sauce** 2. Crême sauce

Part 4: Nontraditional Sauces

Complete the following statements about nontraditional sauces.

14. Beurre blanc is the name of a sauce composed almost entirely of **butter**.
15. Broken butter sauces are basically just **melted butter**. (two words)
16. Beurre noisette is the French name for browned butter finished with **lemon juice**. (two words)
17. Chutneys are similar to relishes, but use different **spices**.
18. Salsas tend to be spicy hot due to the **chiles** from which they are made.

25

Soups

Terminology

Chapter 25

Activity A

Name ______________________

Date __________ **Period** __________

Circle the clue in parentheses that best completes each of the following statements.

1. The coagulated mixture of ground meat, vegetables, and egg whites that floats on top of stock during the clarifying process is called a (**raft**) (**bisque**) (**consommé**).
2. (**Raft**) (**Clearmeat**) (**Chowder**) is an American seafood-based soup that is flavored with dairy product, bacon, and potato.
3. A mixture of ground meat, vegetables, and egg whites added to stock is called a (**raft**) (**clearmeat**) (**bisque**).
4. (**Raft**) (**Clearmeat**) (**Bisque**) is seafood-based soup that is traditionally thickened with rice and flavored with sherry and brandy.
5. Due to the addition of cream and butter, (**purée**) (**cream**) (**bisque**) soups tend to be the richest and silkiest of soups.
6. (**Purée**) (**Cream**) (**Bisque**) soups are thickened using a purée of well-cooked ingredients.
7. A (**purée**) (**cream**) (**consommé**) soup is unique from other soups because it is made by clarifying stock.
8. Clearmeat that has been coagulated by albumin from egg white and is floating along with trapped impurities on top of stock is called a (**purée**) (**consommé**) (**raft**).
9. (**Purée**) (**Clearmeat**) (**Consommé**) is a perfectly transparent and intensely flavored soup.
10. Often considered a luxury, (**purée**) (**cream**) (**bisque**) soup is often flavored with sherry, tinted red with tomato product, and fortified with cream.
11. Starchy foods such as legumes, potatoes, winter squashes, or rice are often the ingredients of a (**purée**) (**consommé**) (**bisque**) soup.
12. (**Purée**) (**Chowder**) (**Cream**) soups tend to be filling soups that were traditionally made and consumed by fishermen.
13. A soup that consists of milk or stock, thickened with both flour and puréed ingredients, and often finished with cream is a (**purée**) (**clearmeat**) (**cream**) soup.

Comparing Soup Categories

Chapter 25 **Name** ____________________

Activity B **Date** __________ **Period** __________

Read each statement below. Circle the letter *T* if the statement is true. If the statement is false, circle *F* and write the corrected statement on the lines that follow.

T (F) 1. Clear soups are divided into purée soups, cream soups, and bisques and chowders.

Thick soups are divided into purée soups, cream soups, and bisques and chowders.

T (F) 2. Broth soup is unique from other soups because it is made by clarifying stock.

Consommé is unique from other soups because it is made by clarifying stock.

(T) F 3. Thick soups have a round mouthfeel because they are thickened.

T (F) 4. Minestrone, vegetable, and chicken noodle soups are examples of bisque soups.

Minestrone, vegetable, and chicken noodle soups are examples of broth soups.

(T) F 5. When consommé is finished cooking, it must be ladled out of the pot because pouring could break the raft and ruin the consommé.

T (F) 6. After cooking, broth soup should be strained through a coffee filter or cheesecloth.

After cooking, consommé should be strained through a coffee filter or cheesecloth.

T (F) 7. Cream soups are made from thickened milk, never from stock.

Cream soups are made from thickened milk or stock.

(Continued)

Activity B *(Continued)* **Name** ____________________

T F 8. Purée soups get their thickening power from the starchy ingredients in the soup.

____

____

T F 9. Clear soups are thin, generally transparent, and have no vegetables or meat in them.

Clear soups are thin, generally transparent, and often have vegetables

or meat in them.

T F 10. Clear soups are divided into broth soups and consommés.

____

____

Reviewing Key Concepts

Chapter 25 Name ____________________

Activity C Date __________ Period __________

Part 1: Specialty Soups

Circle the clue in parentheses that best completes each of the following statements.

1. Soups classically grouped under the heading of specialty soups are (**traditional soups to which chefs have added a personal touch**) (**soups that cannot be classified as clear or thick**).
2. A beet and red cabbage soup is a popular specialty cold soup called (**vichyssoise**) (**borscht**) (**gazpacho**).
3. A cold cream of potato leek soup is a popular specialty cold soup called (**vichyssoise**) (**borscht**) (**gazpacho**).
4. A Spanish soup of puréed tomatoes, red peppers, garlic, and cucumber is a popular specialty cold soup called (**vichyssoise**) (**borscht**) (**gazpacho**).

Part 2: The Role of Soup Garnishes

Complete the following statements in the space provided.

5. Adding a garnish to a finished soup adds visual appearance, texture, and ____ flavor ____.
6. Garnishes should be bite-sized pieces or smaller because ____ excessively large garnishes are difficult to eat easily ____.
7. Garnishes should be tender because ____ crunchy garnishes are unpleasant in most soups ____.
8. Fatty or oily garnishes should be avoided for consommés because ____ nothing should be added that could cloud the consommé ____.
9. Garnishes should complement the soup in style and ____ flavor ____.
10. The guideline for temperature of soup garnishes is that garnishes for hot soups should be served ____ hot ____ and garnishes for cold soups should be served ____ cold ____.

Activity C *(Continued)* **Name** ____________________________

Part 3: Serving Soups

Circle the clue in parentheses that best completes each of the following statements.

11. To serve a successful hot soup, the temperature of the soup must be (**boiling**) (**slightly warmer than lukewarm**) (**very hot**).
12. To serve a successful cold soup, the temperature of the soup must be (**cool**) (**slightly cooler than room temperature**) (**very cold**).
13. When serving soup, the serving container should be (**the same temperature as the soup**) (**lukewarm for both hot and cold soups**) (**slightly chilled for both hot and cold soups**).
14. An advantage of using a soup plate rather than a soup bowl is that (**soup plates keep hot soup hotter and cold soup cooler**) (**soup plates make a beautiful presentation**).
15. An advantage of using a soup bowl rather than a soup plate is that (**bowls offer a more traditional appearance**) (**soup tends to slosh out or onto the sides of the plate**).
16. Soup should always be served (**in front of the customer**) (**as soon as it is portioned**).

Notes

Vegetable Identification

26

Identifying Common Fresh Vegetables

Chapter 26

Activity A

Name ____________________

Date __________ Period __________

Part 1

First, complete any partial terms. Place a word in each space to complete the name of the vegetable. Next, place the letter of each vegetable in its correct category in the chart.

Categories of Vegetables		
Cabbages D, H, R, V, W	**Fruit Vegetables** J, L, AA	**Greens** Y, Z
Legumes M, N, T, CC	**Mushrooms** Q	**Onions** P, X
Root Vegetables C, I, O, S, BB	**Seeds** K	**Squashes, Winter** A, F, U
Squashes, Summer DD	**Squashes, Other**	**Stalks and Shoots** B, G

A. acorn squash

B. asparagus

C. beets

D. broccoli

E. broccoli rabe

F. butternut squash

G. cardoons

H. cauliflower

I. celery root

J. chile peppers

K. corn

L. eggplant

M. French beans

N. green beans

O. jicama

P. leeks

Q. morels

R. napa cabbage

S. parsnips

T. peas

U. pumpkins

V. red cabbage

W. savoy cabbage

X. shallots

Y. spinach

Z. Swiss chard

AA. tomatoes

BB. turnips

CC. wax beans

DD. yellow squash

(Continued)

Activity A *(Continued)* **Name** ______________________

Part 2

First, complete any partial terms. Place a word in each space to complete the name of the vegetable. Next, place the letter of each vegetable in its correct category in the chart.

Categories of Vegetables		
Cabbages E, P	**Fruit Vegetables** B, EE ,FF	**Greens** J, Q, T, HH
Legumes C, D, L, O, R, S, U, V, X, AA, DD	**Mushrooms** F, Y, GG	**Onion** N, BB, CC
Root Vegetables G, Z	**Seeds**	**Squashes, Winter**
Squashes, Summer W, II, JJ	**Squashes, Other** I, K	**Stalks and Shoots** A, H, M

A. artichokes
B. avocado
C. black beans
D. black-eyed peas
E. Brussels sprouts
F. button mushroom
G. carrots
H. celery
I. chayote
J. collard greens
K. cucumbers
L. fava beans
M. fennel
N. garlic
O. Great Northern beans
P. green cabbage
Q. kale
R. lentils
S. lima beans
T. mustard greens
U. navy beans
V. okra
W. patty pan
X. pinto beans
Y. portobello mushroom
Z. radishes
AA. red kidney beans
BB. red onion
CC. scallions
DD. soybeans
EE. sweet peppers
FF. tomatillos
GG. truffles
HH. turnip greens
II. yellow squash
JJ. zucchini

Selecting Vegetables

Chapter 26 Name ____________________

Activity B Date ____________ Period ____________

Part 1: Recognizing Quality Factors in Vegetables

Read each statement below. Circle the letter *T* if the statement is true. If the statement is false, circle *F* and write the corrected statement on the lines that follow.

T (F) 1. Extra large cucumbers with a yellowish color are the best choice for cucumbers.

Extra large cucumbers with a yellowish color are overmature.

T (F) 2. Soft onions that are beginning to sprout are the best choice.

Hard onions with dry crackly skins and no sprouts are the best choice.

(T) F 3. Quality asparagus has tight tips, straight stalks, and no more than an inch of woody base at the bottom of the stalk.

T (F) 4. The best quality greens may have yellow spots.

The best quality greens have crisp leaves with solid green color and no yellow or brown spots.

T (F) 5. Choose cabbage that has enough space between leaves for the head to breathe.

Choose cabbages with firm, tightly packed heads and crisp leaves.

(T) F 6. Carrots should not have green shoulders and should break with a snap when bent.

T (F) 7. Broccoli rabe is known for its pronounced, sweet flavor.

Broccoli rabe is known for its pronounced flavor that many consider bitter.

(Continued)

Activity B *(Continued)* **Name** ____________________

T (F) 8. The caps of button mushrooms should be white and the gills should be dark and open.

The caps of button mushrooms should be tight and closed showing none of the dark gills underneath.

T (F) 9. Choose corn with small kernels, dry silk, and a green husk.

Choose corn with good size, closely packed kernels; moist silk; and a green husk.

T (F) 10. Eggplant should have a firm texture and dull skin.

Eggplants should have a soft texture and shiny skin that is free from blemishes.

Part 2: Fresh Vegetables in Season

For each vegetable listed, circle the choice that best describes its availability or peak season. Some answers may include more than one season.

Vegetable	Season (circle all that apply)				
Root vegetables are at their peak during	spring	summer	**(fall**	**winter)**	year-round
Cabbages are available	spring	summer	fall	winter	**(year-round)**
Broccoli is available	spring	summer	fall	winter	**(year-round)**
Asparagus peaks	**(spring)**	summer	fall	winter	year-round
Fresh morel mushrooms are available	**(spring)**	summer	fall	winter	year-round
Wax beans are available	spring	**(summer)**	fall	winter	year-round
Cauliflower is available	spring	summer	fall	winter	**(year-round)**
Zucchini is fresh	spring	**(summer)**	fall	winter	year-round
Cardoons are ready	spring	summer	**(fall**	**winter)**	year-round
Pattypan is fresh	spring	**(summer)**	fall	winter	year-round
Green beans are available	spring	summer	fall	winter	**(year-round)**
Italian beans are available	spring	**(summer)**	fall	winter	year-round
Fresh chanterelle mushrooms are available	spring	**(summer**	**fall)**	winter	year-round
Truffles are harvested in	spring	summer	fall	**(winter)**	year-round
French beans are available	spring	summer	fall	winter	**(year-round)**

Reviewing Key Concepts

Chapter 26 Name ______________________________

Activity C Date ____________Period____________

Part 1: Purchase Forms of Vegetables

Describe the common purchase forms of packaging for the following fresh vegetables. There may be more than one form of packaging.

1. Dry onions: 50-pound (22 kg) mesh sacks or cardboard cases, or 25-pound (11 kg) sacks
2. Beets without tops: 25-pound bags
3. Bunch spinach: 20- to 22-pound (9 to 10 kg) wooden crates containing 24 bunches
4. Asparagus: crates of 15 or 30 pounds (7 or 14 kg)
5. Standard cucumbers: 50- to 55-pound (22 to 25 kg) bushel cartons or smaller 24-count baskets
6. Regular tomatoes: sorted by size and packed in a two-layer, 20-pound (9 kg) case
7. French beans: 5-pound (2 kg) cases
8. Button mushrooms: 10-pound (4.5 kg) baskets

Activity C *(Continued)* **Name** ______________________________

Part 2: Processing and Grading Vegetables

Circle the clue in parentheses that best completes each of the following statements.

9. Processed vegetables include **(only canned vegetables) (only frozen vegetables) (both canned and frozen vegetables)**.
10. Canned vegetables are **(more) (less)** consistent in quality and yield than fresh vegetables.
11. Green vegetables are more likely to lose their color when **(canned) (frozen)**.
12. Canned vegetables are **(more) (less)** expensive than fresh vegetables.
13. Canned vegetables often have a slightly different flavor and appearance than their fresh counterparts because they are **(inferior quality) (cooked during the canning process)**.
14. Frozen vegetables are (**less**) **(more)** expensive than canned vegetables.
15. Cooking time for frozen vegetables is often (**more**) **(less)** than for fresh vegetables.
16. The USDA has a (**mandatory**) **(voluntary)** grading system for both fresh and processed vegetables.
17. For most fresh vegetables, the top grade is either No. 1 or (**Extra Standard**) **(Fancy)**.
18. For canned or frozen vegetables, the grades are US Grade A or (**Extra Standard**) (**Standard**) **(Fancy)**; US Grade B or **(Extra Standard)** (**Fancy**) (**Standard**); US Grade C or **(Standard)** (**Fancy**) (**Extra Standard**).
19. When grading processed vegetables, the product is scored on its character, color, (**firmness**) (**attractiveness**) **(uniformity of size)**, and absence of defects.
20. Heat in chile peppers is measured in (**ancho**) **(Scoville heat units)** (**capsaicin**).

Vegetable Cookery

27

Terminology

Chapter 27 Name ______________________

Activity A Date ____________ Period ____________

Circle the clue in parentheses that best completes each of the following statements.

1. The process of plunging vegetables into ice water after cooking is called (**blanching**) (**glazing**) (**shocking**).
2. (**Cellulose**) (**Al dente**) (**Blanching**) literally means "to the tooth." This term is used to describe food that is cooked to the point that it (**gives some slight resistance to the tooth**) (**requires no actual chewing**).
3. In cooking, the process of giving something a shiny coating is called (**blanching**) (**glazing**) (**shocking**).
4. The rigid tissue of plants is composed mainly of microscopic fibers called (**cellulose**) (**al dente**) (**chlorophyll**).
5. The purpose of shocking is to (**preserve color**) (**stop the cooking process**) (**allow vegetables to absorb liquid**).
6. The process of partially cooking an item in rapidly boiling water is called (**blanching**) (**glazing**) (**shocking**).
7. Vegetables cooked al dente are (**crunchy**) (**mushy**) (**neither mushy nor crunchy**).
8. The human digestive system is unable to break down (**cellulose**) (**al dente**) (**chlorophyll**).
9. The chemical that gives green vegetables their color is (**cellulose**) (**al dente**) (**chlorophyll**).
10. Chefs use a sauce, reduced stock, or a process similar to sautéing for (**blanching**) (**glazing**) (**shocking**) vegetables.
11. In addition to seasoning vegetables, adding salt during cooking also helps preserve the (**cellulose**) (**al dente**) (**chlorophyll**) in the vegetables.

How Does Cooking Affect Vegetables?

Chapter 27 **Name** ______________________

Activity B **Date** __________ **Period** __________

Read each statement below. Circle the letter *T* if the statement is true. If the statement is false, circle *F* and write the corrected statement on the lines that follow.

(T) F 1. Cooking breaks down cellulose in vegetables, making the texture more appealing and easier to digest.

T (F) 2. The pH of the liquid used to cook vegetables affects their color. The pigments of yellow-orange vegetables are most affected.

The pH of the liquid used to cook vegetables affects their color. The pigments of yellow-orange vegetables are least affected.

T (F) 3. Cooking affects the texture of vegetables. Established cooking times are not always reliable so chefs test vegetables at the thinnest part to see if they are properly cooked.

Cooking affects the texture of vegetables. Established cooking times are not always reliable so chefs test vegetables at the thickest most fibrous part to see if they are properly cooked.

T (F) 4. The colors of red, white, and green vegetables are enhanced by being cooked in an acidic solution.

The colors of red and white vegetables are enhanced by being cooked in an acidic solution; however, green vegetables' colors are enhanced by cooking in an alkaline solution.

(T) F 5. Nutrients in vegetables can become dissolved in cooking water.

(Continued)

Activity B ***(Continued)*** **Name** ______________________

T (F) 6. A slightly alkaline solution preserves the color in red and white vegetables.

A slightly acidic solution preserves the color in red and white vegetables.

(T) F 7. Chefs try to limit the time vegetables are exposed to air, light, and heat in order to retain nutrients as much as possible.

T (F) 8. To achieve proper texture, chefs determine cooking method and length of cooking time based on the amount of chlorophyll in vegetables.

To achieve proper texture, chefs determine cooking method and length of cooking time based on the amount of cellulose in vegetables.

T (F) 9. Adding baking soda to cooking water for green vegetables helps preserve their green color as well as their texture and nutrients.

Adding baking soda to cooking water for green vegetables helps preserve their green color but destroys their texture and nutrients.

T (F) 10. Cooking preserves the properties of natural sugars in vegetables and keeps them from caramelizing.

During cooking, the natural sugars present in the vegetables can be caramelized.

(T) F 11. The gratiner method combines béchamel-based sauces, cheese, or bread crumbs to create a browned surface on vegetable dishes.

T (F) 12. Add salt and such acidic ingredients as tomatoes at the beginning of the simmering time to give dried beans and lentils a tender texture.

Add salt and acidic ingredients near the end of cooking time to give dried beans and lentils a tender texture.

Cooking Vegetables

Chapter 27 **Name** ______________________________

Activity C **Date** ____________**Period**____________

Part 1: Parcooking

Circle the clue in parentheses that best completes each of the following statements.

1. Parcooking vegetables saves time during busy service periods, allows vegetables to be finished a variety of ways, allows vegetables with different textures and colors to be properly cooked when served together, and gives better control **(of nutrients)** **(over the cooking process)** **(of flavors)**.

2. Blanching is done as quickly as possible to preserve (**texture and color**) (**color and nutrients**) (**texture, color, and nutrients**).

3. To blanch vegetables properly, add them to water that is (**cool**) (**almost simmering**) (**rapidly boiling**).

4. Once vegetables are blanched to correct doneness, you should stop the cooking process by shocking which involves (**turning off heat and setting pan aside**) (**plunging vegetables into ice water and letting them sit**) (**plunging vegetables into ice water and immediately draining them**).

Part 2: Finishing Techniques

On the space provided before each of the statements below, write *sautéing*, *glazing*, or *gratiner* to indicate the type of finishing method being described.

glazing 5. Vegetables are tossed with butter and a sweet syrupy ingredient that adds both flavor and a glossy shine.

sautéing 6. Vegetables are placed in a sauteuse and quickly tossed over moderate heat with whole butter, salt, and pepper.

glazing 7. This technique works best with vegetables that are complemented by a sweet flavoring, such as root vegetables.

gratiner 8. Béchamel-based sauces, cheese, or bread crumbs are often used to create a browned surface on vegetable dishes under a broiler or salamander; or in a hot oven.

glazing 9. Vegetables are finished with a sauce or reduced stock.

(Continued)

Activity C *(Continued)* **Name** ____________________________

Part 3: Cooking Methods

Circle the clue in parentheses that best completes each of the following statements.

10. Moist-heat cooking methods include (**steaming, stir-frying, and stewing**) (**steaming, stewing, and braising**) (**steaming, grilling, and stewing**).

11. Dry-heat cooking methods include (**stir-frying, deep frying, baking, roasting, braising, and grilling**) (**stir-frying, deep frying, baking, roasting, stewing, and grilling**) (**stir-frying, deep frying, baking, roasting, and grilling**).

12. Vegetables to be (**roasted**) (**deep-fried**) (**stir-fried**) should be cut in small, even pieces for proper cooking.

13. Vegetables are (**steamed**) (**stewed**) (**braised**) by partially covering them with a flavored liquid and then simmering.

14. Vegetables to be (**grilled**) (**braised**) (**deep-fried**) should be cut thick enough so they do not dry out and large enough so they don't fall through the rack.

15. (**Baking and roasting**) (**Stewing and baking**) (**Steaming and stir-frying**) are often done with whole vegetables.

16. Because delicate vegetables such as spinach or pea pods are easy to overcook, (**stir-frying**) (**braising**) (**steaming**) is not a recommended cooking method for these vegetables.

17. Vegetables to be (**roasted**) (**deep-fried**) (**stir-fried**) are coated with a breading or batter before cooking to seal in moisture and keep them from becoming too greasy.

18. Vegetables are braised (**in the oven**) (**on the stove top**) (**on the stove top or in the oven**).

19. The main difference between the stewing and braising processes is the (**vegetables are cut smaller**) (**cooking temperature is higher**) (**lid is kept tighter**) in the stewing process.

20. Because dried beans and lentils require a long simmering time, they should be (**soaked overnight in cold salt water**), (**soaked in warm water an hour the day of cooking**) (**soaked overnight in cold water**) to speed up the cooking time.

Notes

Starch Identification

28

Terminology

Chapter 28 **Name** ______________________________

Activity A **Date** ____________ **Period** ____________

Match the following terms and identifying phrases.

B 1. Any rice sold with the bran layer left attached.

H 2. Not a variety of potato but an immature potato of any variety.

F 3. A rice that has been fully cooked and then freeze-dried.

A 4. The first part of the grain kernel that lies just under the husk and is rich in fiber.

M 5. Rice in which the bran layer has been pearled during the milling process.

G 6. Type of potato that is high in starch and typically used for baked potatoes.

C 7. Rice that has been parboiled to remove surface starch.

J 8. A hard variety of wheat that is a favored pasta ingredient.

E 9. The smallest part of the grain kernel and a source of fat.

D 10. The largest part of the grain kernel.

L 11. Potato that is relatively low in starch and typically used when boiling potatoes.

K 12. The enlarged part of the underground root of potato plants that is eaten.

I 13. The continental landmass of the Americas.

A. bran
B. brown rice
C. converted rice
D. endosperm
E. germ
F. instant rice
G. mealy potato
H. new potato
I. New World
J. semolina
K. tuber
L. waxy potato
M. white rice

Choosing the Right Potato

Chapter 28 Name ______________________

Activity B Date __________ Period __________

Complete the following chart by writing ***mealy, all-purpose, specialty,*** or ***waxy*** to indicate the type of potato each variety is. Answer the questions that follow.

Potato Varieties and Type	
Variety	**Type**
Fingerling	specialty
Long White	all-purpose
Peruvian Blue	specialty
Round Red	waxy
Round White	all-purpose
Russet Burbank	mealy
Yukon Gold	all-purpose

1. Which variety of potato is the best choice for baked potatoes?

   Russet Burbank

2. Which variety of potato is the best choice for boiled potatoes?

   Round Red

3. Which variety of potato is the best choice for frying potatoes?

   Russet Burbank

4. Which variety of the potato might be sold as a new potato?

   Round Reds are commonly used for this purpose, however, any variety of immature potatoes can be sold as new potatoes.

5. Why are sweet potatoes and yams not included in the varieties list above?

   They are botanically different from potatoes.

Recognizing Common Grains and Grain Products

Chapter 28 **Name** ____________________

Activity C **Date** __________ **Period** __________

Part 1

Match the following terms and identifying phrases.

D 1. Coarsely ground hominy, commonly cooked as a hot cereal and often served with breakfast in the southern United States.

F 2. Finely milled flour made from hominy. Use to make the outside coating for tamales.

G 3. Noodles made from rice flour.

B 4. The only grain native to the America's.

I 5. A variety of wheat favored as a pasta ingredient because its texture allows pasta to stay firmer for longer.

J 6. The most important of the five grains that have fed Western civilization for the last 12,000 years.

E 7. Whole kernels of corn that have been treated with lye. Can be served as a side dish or an ingredient in soups and stews.

H 8. Primarily used as a flavoring in fermented beverages and bread products.

A 9. One of the oldest grains eaten by people. Today, most is used to make beer or animal feed, but a pearled version is used in soups and stews.

K 10. Not a true rice but the seed from a water plant that grows in the upper United States. Has a nutty flavor when cooked.

C 11. Fine pasta-like product made from hard durum wheat. Can be steamed or cooked in a liquid and is traditionally served in North Africa with stews.

A. barley
B. corn
C. couscous
D. grits
E. hominy
F. masa harina
G. rice noodles
H. rye
I. semolina
J. wheat
K. wild rice

Activity C *(Continued)* **Name** ______________________

Part 2

Match the following terms and identifying phrases.

E 1. Made by milling a special type of corn into different size grinds. Used for coating fried products, in breads, and as a cooked cereal called mush.

L 2. A medium-sized, round tube of pasta.

C 3. Also called *soba*, is popular in Japan. Used hot in soup or cold with a dipping sauce.

N 4. Most often cooked in liquid and eaten as hot oatmeal, but also added to breads.

G 5. Popular Asian noodle also called wheat noodles. Typically served in soups or fried crisp and served as a pancake or used to garnish.

Q 6. Pasta shaped like a wagon wheel, often used in soups or pasta salad.

A 7. Long, thin, delicate pasta also called fidelini.

I 8. Long, twisted shaped pasta served with a sauce or broken and added to soup or salad.

M 9. Was a staple of the Chinese diet before rice. Typically boiled into porridge.

B 10. Noodles made from bean starch and prepared in ways similar to rice noodles.

S 11. Whole wheat kernels without the hull. Good source of dietary fiber.

J 12. Long, flat pasta that is typically used in casseroles.

R 13. The favorite pasta in the United States.

F 14. A finely milled corn flour used as a coating or a thickening agent for hot liquids.

T 15. A small tube pasta often used for baked dishes and pasta salads.

P 16. The seed of a grass plant grown in flooded fields called paddies.

H 17. Long, flat pasta about ¼ inch (1 cm) wide. It is served with a variety of sauces.

D 18. Made by removing the bran layer from wheat and then steaming and drying the product. Can be ground into different textures and soaked in water to be eaten raw or cooked.

K 19. Long pasta about 3/16 inch (0.5 cm) wide.

O 20. The Italian version of cornmeal. Used to prepare Italian side dish or entrée.

A. angel hair
B. bean starch noodles
C. buckwheat noodles
D. bulgur
E. cornmeal
F. cornstarch
G. egg noodles
H. fettucini
I. fusilli
J. lasagna
K. linguine
L. manicotti
M. millet
N. oats
O. polenta
P. rice
Q. rotelle
R. spaghetti
S. wheat berries
T. ziti

Starch Cookery

29

Terminology

Chapter 29

Activity A

Name ______________________________

Date ____________**Period**____________

Circle the clue in parentheses that best completes each of the following statements.

1. The term *gaufrette* describes a (**tool for cutting potatoes into a waffle shape**) (**classification of deep-fried potatoes**) (**technique to increase the water content of potatoes before panfrying**).
2. If the recipe calls for cooking pasta al dente, you should continue cooking until the pasta is fully cooked (**and soft and mushy**) (**but not soft and mushy**) (**and crispy**).
3. To rehydrate a product, you must (**add water back to**) (**remove a quantity of water from**) the product.
4. A rice dish cooked at an active simmer while being stirred is (**risotto**) (**pilaf**).
5. A cooking method that includes sautéing the grain in hot fat, then adding hot liquid and simmering without stirring is (**risotto**) (**pilaf**).
6. (**Risotto**) (**Pilaf**) (**Al dente**) is a cooking method, as well as, the name of a traditional Italian rice dish.
7. A mandolin is typically used to prepare (**gaufrette**) (**al dente**) (**rehydrate**) potatoes.
8. Dry pasta requires a longer cooking time than fresh or fresh frozen pasta because cooking also acts to (**rehydrate**) (**al dente**) the pasta.
9. The (**boiling**) (**pilaf**) method is different from simmering because the aromatics are sweated and the grains of rice are coated with the fat before liquid is added.
10. "To the tooth" is a phrase used to describe pasta cooked (**al dente**) (**rehydrate**).
11. Pilaf can be traced back to (**Southeast Asia**) (**Persia/Iran**) (**Egypt**).

Calculating Rice to Liquid Ratio

Chapter 29 Name ______________________

Activity B Date __________ Period__________

Use the table below to answer the questions that follow. Write your answers in the spaces provided. Include the unit of measure in your answers. For metric answers, round up to the nearest whole number.

Rice to Liquid Ratios	
Rice Type	**Parts Liquid to 1 Part Rice (by volume)**
Arborio	3
Basmati	1½ to 2
Brown, long-grain	2½ to 3
Converted	1¾ to 2
White, long-grain	1½ to 2
White, medium-grain	1½ to 1¾
White, short-grain	1½ to 1¾

Use the ratios in the table above to calculate an equal ratio consisting of different quantities. To calculate ratios when one of the quantities is unknown, you can find it by cross multiplying.

Example: You need to cook 4 cups of long-grain brown rice. If you use the minimum amount of liquid, how much will you need? First, write the ratio for minimum liquid to long-grain brown rice from the table above.

2½:1

Convert the fraction to a decimal for ease of use and write the ratio in the form of a division problem.

$$\frac{\mathbf{2.5}\ \text{cups liquid}}{\mathbf{1}\ \text{cup rice}}$$

Set up the problem to solve for the unknown (*n*) cups of liquid (in this case the "parts" are measured in cups).

$$\frac{2.5}{1} = \frac{n}{4}$$

Activity B *(Continued)* **Name** ______________________

Use cross multiplication to solve for the unknown amount of liquid or rice.

$$\frac{2.5}{1} \times \frac{n}{4}$$

$$1 \times n = 2.5 \times 4$$

$$n = 10 \text{ cups liquid}$$

Check your work by substituting your solution for the unknown *n*.

$$\frac{2.5}{1} \times \frac{10}{4}$$

$$2.5 \times 4 = 1 \times 10$$

$$10 = 10$$

1. How much liquid do you need to cook 1 cup of arborio rice? 3 cups
2. How much liquid do you need to cook 250 mL of converted rice?

range is 438–500 mL; $\frac{1.75}{1} = \frac{n}{250 \text{ mL}}$ $n = 438$ mL

and $\frac{2}{1} = \frac{n}{250 \text{ mL}}$ $n = 500$ mL

3. What is the amount of arborio rice you can cook in 8 cups of liquid?

$$\frac{3}{1} = \frac{8 \text{ cups}}{n}$$

2⅔ cups; $3 \times n = 8 \times 1$

$$3n = 8$$

$$n = \frac{8}{3}$$

$n = 2.66$ cups or 2⅔ cups

4. What is the minimum amount of liquid needed to cook 1 cup of white, medium-grain rice?

1½ cups

(Continued)

Activity B (*Continued)* **Name** ____________________________

5. What is the minimum amount of liquid needed to cook 500 mL of white, long-grain rice?

750 mL;

$$\frac{1.5}{1} = \frac{n}{500\text{ mL}}$$

$$1.5 \times 500 = 1 \times n$$

$$n = 750\text{ mL}$$

6. What is the maximum amount of liquid needed to cook 500 mL of white, long-grain rice? ____________________________

1000 mL or 1 L;

$$\frac{2}{1} = \frac{n}{500\text{ mL}}$$

$$2 \times 500 = 1 \times n$$

$$n = 1000\text{ mL} = 1\text{ L}$$

7. Which two types of rice require the greatest liquid to grain ratio?
arborio and long-grain brown rice

8. How much liquid do you need to cook 3 cups of arborio rice?

9 cups;

$$\frac{3}{1} = \frac{n}{3\text{ cups}}$$

$$3 \times 3 = 1 \times n$$

$$n = 9\text{ cups}$$

9. How much liquid do you need to cook ½ cup of arborio rice?

1½ cups;

$$\frac{3}{1} = \frac{n}{0.5\text{ cups}}$$

$$3 \times 0.5 = 1 \times n$$

$$n = 1.5\text{ cups} = 1\tfrac{1}{2}\text{ cups}$$

10. You have 2 cups of broth and want to use all of it as the liquid to cook a batch of rice. You have exactly 1 cup of each of the types of rice listed in the table. To use a proper grain to liquid ratio, which type(s) of rice could you choose to cook in your broth?
basmati, converted, long-grain white

Reviewing Key Concepts

Chapter 29 **Name** ____________________

Activity C **Date** __________ **Period** __________

Part 1: Cooking Potatoes

Complete each statement below by filling in the missing word or words.

1. The four most common methods for cooking potatoes are ___baking___, ___boiling___, ___sautéing/panfrying___ and ___deep-frying___.

2. Potatoes are generally classified as being either ___mealy___ or ___waxy___.

3. The cooking methods that work best for ___mealy___ potatoes, commonly called baking potatoes, are ___baking___ and ___frying___.

4. The most common method of cooking ___waxy___ potatoes, commonly called boiling potatoes, is ___boiling___.

5. Bake potatoes in a ___350___ to ___400___ degree oven until done. You can test to see if a baking potato is done by ___how easily a paring knife can pierce it___.

6. Most deep-fried potatoes must be cooked in two stages. First, heat oil to ___250___°F (___120___°C) and deep-fry for ___2___ to ___3___ minutes. Then heat oil to___350___°F (___180___°C) and deep-fry until golden brown and cooked internally.

Part 2: Cooking Grains

Match the following terms and identifying phrases.

___B___ 7. Sauté grain in hot fat, then add hot liquid; simmer grain without stirring.

___C___ 8. Keep rice at an active simmer while stirring; continually add hot seasoned liquid in small amounts until rice is tender.

___A___ 9. Add the grain to a large amount of lightly salted boiling water.

___D___ 10. Simmer a measured amount of grain in a measured amount of liquid in a covered pot for the appropriate time for the grain.

A. boiling
B. pilaf
C. risotto
D. simmering

(Continued)

Activity C ***(Continued)*** **Name** ______________________

Part 3: Cooking Pasta

Summarize the four steps for cooking pasta in the space provided.

Step 1 **Bring one gallon (3.8 L) of lightly salted water (2 to 3 Tbsp.) per pound of pasta to a boil.**

Step 2 **Add pasta and stir to separate the pieces of pasta.**

Step 3 **Cook pasta at a rolling boil until al dente.**

Step 4 **Drain pasta immediately and serve.**

Meat and Poultry Identification

30

Terminology

Chapter 30 **Name** ______________________

Activity A **Date** __________ **Period** __________

Match the following terms and identifying phrases.

L 1. When muscle tissue temporarily becomes extremely hard and stiff.

D 2. A flexible but tough connective tissue found in ligaments and tendons, also called *silver skin*.

A 3. Resting time for meat after slaughter.

H 4. The internal organs and extremities that are removed before an animal or bird is butchered, also called *variety meats*.

F 5. An assurance of safety and wholesomeness, not an indication of quality.

J 6. An evaluation of traits related to tenderness, juiciness, and flavor.

I 7. A major division of the carcass.

B 8. The most prevalent connective tissue in meats.

G 9. Intramuscular fat.

M 10. The loss of water during the cooking process.

C 11. Protein that bundles muscle tissue together and connects muscle to bones, joints, and skin.

E 12. The offal meats commonly from poultry.

K 13. To extract fat by melting.

N 14. An evaluation of the amount of lean, closely trimmed boneless cuts a carcass will produce.

A. aging
B. collagen
C. connective tissue
D. elastin
E. giblets
F. inspection
G. marbling
H. offal
I. primal cut
J. quality grade
K. render
L. rigor mortis
M. shrinkage
N. yield grade

Reviewing Key Concepts

Chapter 30 | **Name** ______________________

Activity B | **Date** __________ **Period** __________

Part 1: Meat Composition

On the space provided before each of the characteristics, write ***muscle, connective tissue,*** or ***fat*** to indicate the component of meat being described.

connective tissue 1. Is the most important factor in determining the toughness of a cut of meat.

fat 2. Provides moisture, tenderness, and flavor to meats.

muscle 3. Is the most important part of meat.

fat 4. Two types are subcutaneous and intramuscular.

connective tissue 5. Two types are elastin and collagen.

muscle 6. Cutting across the grain of this component creates a tender finished product.

Part 2: Aging

Circle the clue in parentheses that best completes each of the following statements.

7. While meat is in the **(rigor mortis)** **(dry aging)** **(wet aging)** stage, it is difficult to cut and extremely tough to eat.

8. The traditional method for aging meat is the **(rigor mortis)** **(dry aging)** **(wet aging)** process.

9. The process that ages meat while in vacuum-sealed plastic bags is the **(rigor mortis)** **(dry aging)** **(wet aging)** process.

10. **(Rigor mortis)** **(Dry aging)** **(Wet aging)** involves hanging meat in a low humidity refrigerator for as long as six weeks.

11. The **(rigor mortis)** **(dry aging)** **(wet aging)** process is a more cost effective aging method because there is reduced loss due to dry, moldy meat.

12. **(Marbling)** **(Enzymes)** **(Fats)** in meats cause muscle tissues to relax and even break down connective tissue.

(Continued)

Activity B ***(Continued)*** **Name** ______________________

Part 3: Selecting a Cooking Process

Read each statement below. Circle the letter *T* if the statement is true. If the statement is false, circle *F* and write the corrected statement on the lines that follow.

T (F) 12. The most important consideration when trying to match the best cooking method for a cut of meat is the amount of fat in the meat.

The most important consideration when trying to match the best cooking method for a cut of meat is the amount of connective tissue in the meat.

(T) F 13. Cuts of meat from the shoulder section of an animal are best simmered, braised, or stewed because these cuts are usually less tender.

____

____

T (F) 14. Tender cuts are best cooked by moist methods.

Tender cuts are best cooked by dry methods.

T (F) 15. Cuts from along the back of an animal are best when simmered, braised, or stewed.

Cuts from along the back of an animal are best when roasted, grilled, or sautéed.

Part 4: Inspection and Grading

Circle the clue in parentheses that best completes each of the following statements.

16. (Grading) **((Inspection))** is an assurance of safety and wholesomeness and not an indication of quality.
17. **((Grading))** (Inspection) is classifying products according to quality.
18. **((Grading))** (Inspection) identifies the qualities that affect the tenderness and flavor of meat and poultry.
19. (Grading) **((Inspection))** is mandatory.
20. **((Grading))** (Inspection) is voluntary.
21. (Grading) **((Inspection))** is performed on live animals before slaughter and includes examination of animals' organs after slaughter.
22. **((Grading))** (Inspection) of meats is based on marbling, maturity, and muscle conformation.
23. **((Grading))** (Inspection) of poultry is based on size, flesh quality, and visible defects.

Foodservice Use of Meats and Poultry

Chapter 30 Name ______________________

Activity C Date __________ Period __________

Part 1: Identifying

Read each statement below. Circle the letter *T* if the statement is true. If the statement is false, circle *F* and write the corrected statement on the lines that follow.

T (F) 1. There is just one way to cut subprimals regardless of their planned final use.

There are many ways to cut subprimals based on their planned final use.

T (F) 2. Foodservice subprimals are essentially the same as retail cuts sold in supermarkets.

Foodservice subprimals are not the same as retail cuts sold in supermarkets.

T (F) 3. The quality of meat is not affected by the way subprimals are cut and trimmed.

The quality of meat is greatly affected by the way subprimals are cut and trimmed.

(T) F 4. IMPS numbers each identify a specific variation of cutting and trimming subprimals.

T (F) 5. Chefs typically specify meat items by name of cut when ordering from a purveyor.

Chefs typically specify meat items by IMPS number when ordering from a purveyor.

(T) F 6. Muscle tissue constitutes the most important part of meat.

T (F) 7. Amino acids are complex proteins produced by living cells that bring about many different reactions in the body.

Enzymes are complex proteins produced by living cells that bring about many different reactions in the body.

Activity C *(Continued)* Name ____________________

Part 2: Choosing Appropriate Cooking Methods for Meat

Complete the charts below with the primal cut and appropriate cooking method for each of the subprimal cuts of meat.

Beef and Veal		
Primal Cut	**Subprimal Cut**	**Appropriate Cooking Method**
Beef		
chuck	Square Cut Chuck	braise, stew, or used for ground beef
loin	Porterhouse Steak	grill, broil
rib	Rib Eye Roll Steak, boneless	grill, broil
Veal		
rack	Hotel Rack	roast
leg	Cutlets, boneless	sauté

Lamb and Pork		
Primal Cut	**Subprimal Cut**	**Appropriate Cooking Method**
Lamb		
rack	Rack, frenched	roast
Pork		
loin	Tenderloin	roast, grill, sauté

(Continued)

Activity C *(Continued)* **Name** ______________________

Part 3: Choosing Appropriate Cooking Methods for Poultry

Complete the chart below by writing the appropriate cooking method for each poultry type and class.

Poultry		
Type	**Class**	**Appropriate Cooking Method**
Chicken		
	Cornish game hen	**grill, broil, roast, sauté**
	Broiler/fryer	**all methods**
	Capon	**roast, poach**
Turkey		
	Hen	**all methods**
	Tom	**roast**
Duck		
	Duckling	**all methods**
	Roaster	**roast, braise**
Goose		
	Young	**roast**
	Mature	**braise, stew**

Basic Meat and Poultry Preparation

31

Terminology

Chapter 31 **Name** ______________________

Activity A **Date** __________ **Period** __________

Fill in each blank in the letter below with the appropriate culinary term from Chapter 31.

Dear Culinary Hopeful:

You asked about meat and poultry preparation in today's kitchen. Things have changed since the old days when every large food operation had a butcher on staff, who was responsible for all the cutting and trimming of meat items used in the operation. Today's professional kitchens rarely buy an entire animal carcass. However, there is still plenty of cutting and trimming to do. For example, in a process called ___fabrication___, we cut meat or poultry into serving portions. We cut all of our ___steaks___, which is a portion-sized piece cut from a large muscle or group of muscles. This portion may or may not have a bone; but a steak portion called a ___chop___, always has a bone. Another variety, a thin, boneless steak that is prepared by cutting thin slices of a boneless muscle is called a ___cutlet___.

Another part of meat preparation is tying roasts. One of the reasons to tie a large roast is for ___barding___ it, which simply means to cover it with a thin sheet of fat to keep it moist during cooking. Birds to be roasted whole are also tied. When referring to birds, tying is usually called ___trussing___. This process gives the cooked bird a pleasing appearance and ensures even cooking. Roasting poultry is common, but perhaps the most popular cut of poultry is the boneless chicken breast. In fine dining establishments, we commonly present each lobe of the breast with the first joint of the wing still attached. We call this cut ___airline breast___.

So as you can see, there are still plenty of opportunities for meat preparation in the contemporary professional kitchen.

Master Chef

Reviewing Key Concepts

Chapter 31 **Name** ______________________________

Activity B **Date** ____________**Period**____________

Part 1: Proper Handling and Storage

Circle the clue in parentheses that best completes each of the following statements.

1. Fresh meat and poultry should be stored (**below 30°F to 35°F [-1°C to 2°C]**) (**at 30°F to 35°F [-1°C to 2°C]**) (**above 30°F to 35°F [-1°C to 2°C]**).
2. Film-wrapped, vacuum-packed meats have a refrigerated shelf life of (**several days**) (**several weeks**) (**several months**) when kept in their sealed bags.
3. Meat and poultry should be stored on a tray or sheet pan to keep them (**from dripping on other items**) (**organized for quick location**) (**from warming**).
4. Never store raw meats or poultry (**below**) (**on the same level as**) (**above**) cooked or ready-to-eat items.
5. Sanitize (**major**) (**non-refrigerated**) (**all**) food-contact surfaces when storing meats and poultry.

Part 2: Poultry Fabrication

Circle the clue in parentheses that best completes each of the following statements.

6. To begin to split poultry in half, place the bird on the cutting board with the (**breast**) (**back**) toward you and the tail up. After splitting in half, the bird's backbone (**remains with one portion**) (**is cut away and removed**).
7. To cut poultry halves into quarters, you need to find the natural separation between the (**leg and wing**) (**breast and thigh**) (**leg and thigh**) and cut along that line.
8. Another term for preparing eight-cut portions of poultry is (**double quarter**) (**disjointed**).
9. To eight-cut a bird after quartering, the cut to make on the leg-and-thigh quarter is through the joint connecting the (**thigh and drumstick**) (**thigh and wing**) (**leg and wing**).
10. To eight-cut a bird after quartering, the cut to make on the breast-and-wing quarter is through the joint at the base of the (**breast**) (**leg**) (**wing**).

Reviewing Key Concepts

Chapter 31 **Name** ____________________

Activity C **Date** __________ **Period** __________

Part 1: Common Meat Portions

Circle the clue in parentheses that best completes each of the following statements.

1. A (**steak**) (**chop**) (**cutlet**) (**roast**) is a portion-size piece of meat that is cut from a larger muscle or group of muscles.
2. Both a (**steak**) (**chop**) (**cutlet**) (**roast**) and a (**steak**) (**chop**) (**cutlet**) (**roast**) are types of (**steak**) (**chop**) (**cutlet**) (**roast**).
3. A (**steak**) (**chop**) (**cutlet**) (**roast**) always has a bone.
4. A (**steak**) (**chop**) (**cutlet**) (**roast**) sometimes has a bone.
5. A (**steak**) (**chop**) (**cutlet**) (**roast**) never has a bone.
6. A (**steak**) (**chop**) (**cutlet**) (**roast**) is not a portion-size piece of meat.

Part 2: Portioning

Read each statement below. Circle the letter *T* if the statement is true. If the statement is false, circle *F* and write the corrected statement on the lines that follow.

T F 7. Uniformity in portions in the commercial kitchen is measured by appearance.

Uniformity in portions in the commercial kitchen is measured by weight.

T F 8. Consistency in portion size is essential to customer satisfaction and product cost.

T F 9. Small inconsistencies in meat portions are not important but large ones can raise cost.

Any inconsistencies in meat portions are important and can add up to a large amount of money.

(Continued)

Activity C ***(Continued)*** **Name** ______________________

T (F) 10. Most chefs consider portion size variance of more than two ounces (60 g) unacceptable.

Most chefs consider portion size variance of more than one ounce (30 g) unacceptable.

(T) F 11. Many kitchens buy portion-cut meat and poultry rather than deal with cutting portioning themselves.

____

____

Dry-Heat Cooking Methods for Meat and Poultry 32

Terminology

Chapter 32 Name ______________________

Activity A Date __________ Period __________

Match the following terms and identifying phrases. Some terms may be used more than once.

__C__ 1. The process of coating foods with flour.

__F__ 2. The process of browning meat to form an even crust.

__B__ 3. The process that involves simmering pan drippings and liquid to dissolve the drippings.

__C__ 4. When seasoning is added to flour used in this process, the product can be both coated and seasoned in one step.

__A__ 5. The amount of cooking that continues after a large roast is removed from the oven.

__F__ 6. This process does not work properly if the sauté pan is overloaded.

__B__ 7. This process is the first step toward creating a sauce from the pan drippings of a sautéed item.

__E__ 8. The deglazed drippings of a roast that are strained and seasoned.

__A__ 9. Because of this effect, large roasts must be removed in advance of the final desired temperature being reached.

__D__ 10. Thickened jus.

__E__ 11. The French term for *juice*.

__D__ 12. The thickening agent for this product may be roux or a slurry.

A. carryover cooking
B. deglazing
C. dredging
D. gravy
E. jus
F. searing

Comparing Approaches for Roasting

Chapter 32 Name ____________________

Activity B Date __________ Period __________

Complete the concept chart below that compares the two approaches for roasting meats and poultry. Fill in each numbered shape with a phrase from the following list.

At a lower temperature.

Constant heat.

Creates a moist product.

In an oven at one temperature throughout.

More natural juices are lost.

On a range top.

Product might not brown.

Useful for products that won't brown in a short time.

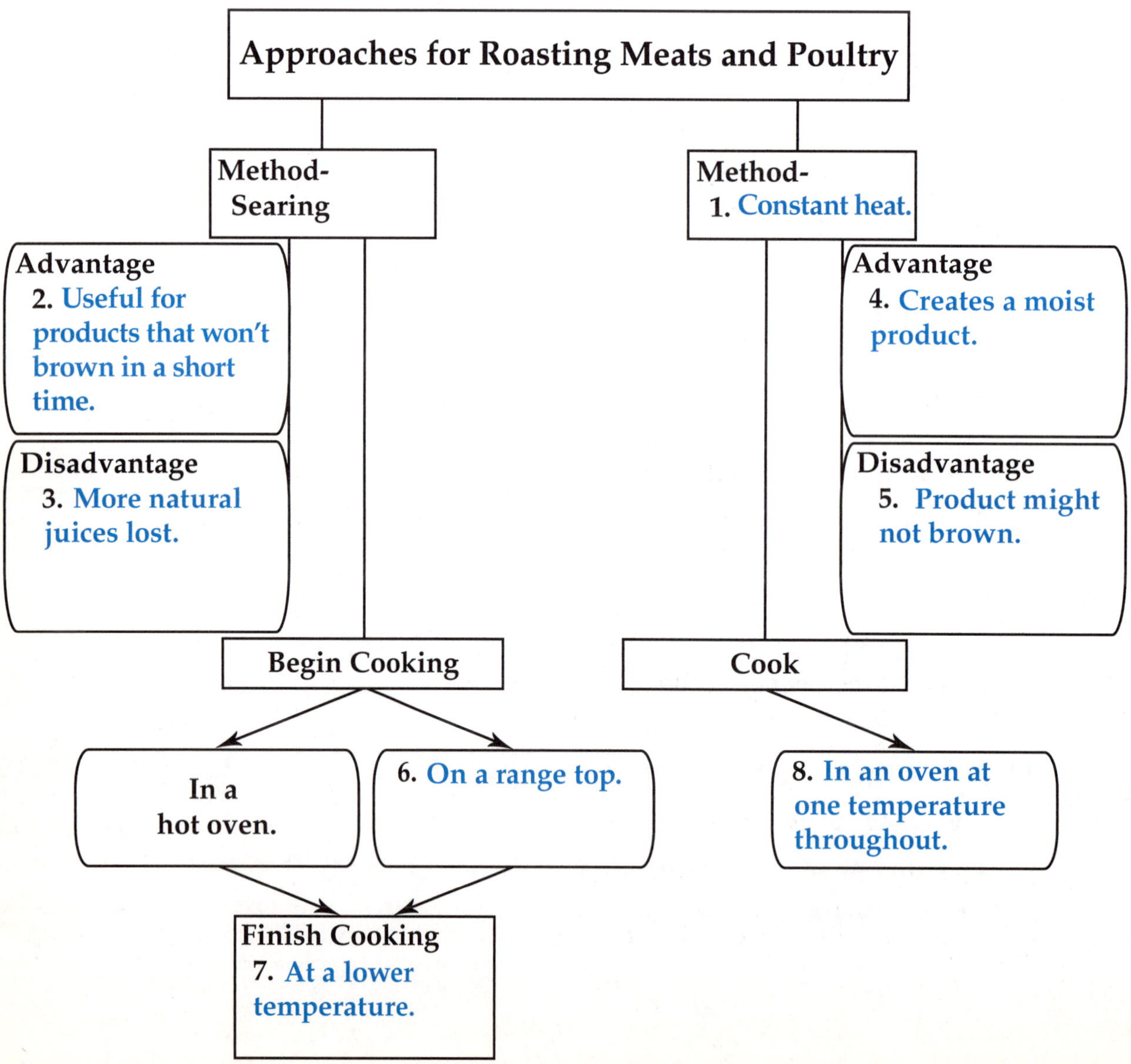

Reviewing Key Concepts

Chapter 32 **Name** ____________________

Activity C **Date** __________ **Period** __________

Part 1: Sautéing and Pan Sauce Preparation

Read each statement below. Circle the letter *T* if the statement is true. If the statement is false, circle *F* and write the corrected statement on the lines that follow.

T (F) 1. Sautéing meat is a quick cooking process done over low heat.

Sautéing meat is a quick cooking process done over high heat.

T (F) 2. To sauté, the fat and product are added to the cold pan.

To sauté, the fat and pan are heated before the product is added.

(T) F 3. A properly sautéed item is evenly seared.

T (F) 4. Any fat is suitable for sautéing.

Fats that do not smoke or burn at high temperatures should be used for sautéing.

(T) F 5. To create a sauce from the drippings left in the sauté pan, the meat must be removed from the pan and liquid must be added.

T (F) 6. The liquid used for deglazing is always water.

Water, stock, wine, or sauce can be used to deglaze.

(Continued)

Activity C *(Continued)* **Name** ______________________

T (F) 7. Sautéing is a good choice for large slices of tougher cuts of meat.

Sautéing is a good choice for small slices of tender cuts of meat.

T (F) 8. When sautéing, fat should be about ¼ inch deep in pan.

When sautéing, fat should just coat the bottom of the pan.

Part 2: Grilling and Broiling

Circle the clue in parentheses that best completes each of the following statements.

9. When (**broiling**) (**grilling**), the heat source is over the meat.
10. When (**broiling**) (**grilling**), the heat source is under the meat.
11. During grilling, drippings create smoke, which (**adds to**) (**has no affect on**) (**detracts from**) the flavor of the meat being cooked.
12. Drippings from (**both broiling and grilling**) (**broiling**) (**grilling**) (**neither broiling nor grilling**) can be used to create sauces.
13. Both the grilling and broiling processes should begin with a (**cold**) (**preheated**) grill or broiler.
14. A clean grill is (**not essential**) (**very important**) to keep food from sticking during grilling.
15. Meat or poultry (**should**) (**should not**) be brushed with oil or butter before grilling or broiling begins.
16. A (**sharp fork**) (**tongs**) should be used to turn or move meat on the grill.
17. Once the meat on a grill starts to sear, rotate it (**30 degrees**) (**45 degrees**) (**90 degrees**) to create cross markings.
18. When broiling thicker pieces of meat or poultry, once the meat is seared it should be finished at a (**higher**) (**constant**) (**lower**) temperature.
19. Testing for doneness by piercing the seared crust of a grilled steak or chop is (**accepted**) (**good**) (**poor**) technique.
20. When testing for doneness, meat that is (**firmer**) (**softer**) will be more well done.
21. Regardless the desired degree of doneness, you must compensate for (**under-cooking**) (**carryover cooking**) (**over-cooking**).

33

Moist-Heat and Combination Cooking Methods for Meat and Poultry

Terminology

Chapter 33 Name ______________________

Activity A Date __________ Period __________

Match the following terms and identifying phrases. Some problems may have more than one correct answer. Some terms may be used more than once.

B 1. Means for determining doneness of larger cuts cooked by simmering or braising.

E 2. Method that applies simmering or braising to bite-size pieces of meat or poultry.

A* 3. Employs the techniques of first searing then cooking in liquid.

C 4. One of its main benefits is the infusion of flavor to the product being cooked.

D** 5. Cooks foods in liquids at temperatures between 185°F and 205°F (85°C–96°C).

A* 6. Is a combination of dry-heat and moist-heat cooking methods.

D, E 7. Enough liquid to fully cover the ingredients is used in this method.

C 8. Cooks foods in liquids at relatively low temperatures between 160°F and 180°F (71°C–82°C).

B 9. Means that when a long-tined fork or skewer is inserted into a cut of cooked meat, the meat easily slides off the fork.

D 10. Cooking method that produces a rich broth.

A. braising
B. fork-tender
C. poaching
D. simmering
E. stewing

*** E could be an additional correct answer because some stews are prepared using braising technique.**
**** A and E could be additional correct answers since these methods both involve simmering.**

Reviewing Key Concepts

Chapter 33 Name ____________

Activity B Date ________ Period ________

Part 1: Poaching

Read each statement below. Circle the letter *T* if the statement is true. If the statement is false, circle *F* and write the corrected statement on the lines that follow.

T (F) 1. Poaching is very important in meat and poultry cookery, but has a limited role with fish.

Poaching is very important in fish cookery, but has a limited role with meat and poultry.

T (F) 2. The main benefit of poaching is its tenderizing effect.

The main benefit of poaching is the infusion of flavor to the product being cooked but has little tenderizing effect.

(T) F 3. Poaching of meat and poultry products is often limited to tender cuts of young poultry, such as the breast.

T (F) 4. Poaching is not a recommended cooking method for sausage.

Poaching is a recommended cooking method for sausage.

(T) F 5. Court bouillon is water flavored with aromatic herbs and mirepoix.

T (F) 6. Stock and vinegar are equally common poaching liquids.

Stock and court bouillon are common poaching liquids.

(Continued)

Activity B ***(Continued)*** **Name** ______________________________

Part 2: Simmering

Circle the clue in parentheses that best completes each of the following statements.

7. Meat and poultry should never be cooked at a boil because extended exposure to the higher temperature causes (**the meat to fall off the bone**) (**the liquid to evaporate**) (**their proteins to toughen**).
8. Simmering (**is the most effective way of breaking down**) (**has little effect on**) (**slows the breaking down of**) collagen.
9. Cuts from the (**forequarter**) (**hindquarter**) of animals and (**mature**) (**immature**) poultry are best cooked by simmering.
10. The means for checking for doneness of large cuts cooked by simmering or braising is called (**firmness**) (**fork-tender**).
11. Collagen is (**limited**) (**abundant**) (**gelatin**) in tough cuts of meat and poultry.
12. The best way to sear meat and poultry for braising is (**with low heat and tomato product**) (**with high heat and stock**) (**with high heat in a small amount of fat on the stovetop**).

Reviewing Key Concepts

Chapter 33 **Name** ____________________

Activity C **Date** __________ **Period** __________

Part 1: Braising

Read each statement below. Circle the letter *T* if the statement is true. If the statement is false, circle *F* and write the corrected statement on the lines that follow.

T (F) 1. Braising is a combination of stewing and poaching cooking methods.

Braising is a combination of dry- and moist-heat cooking methods.

(T) F 2. Braising is used for tough cuts of meat and poultry to make them tender.

T (F) 3. Simmering, unlike braising, begins with searing.

Braising begins with searing, simmering does not.

(T) F 4. Braised dishes are more easily simmered in the oven than on the stove top.

T (F) 5. When braising, add enough liquid to completely cover the meat.

When braising, enough liquid to cover the meat halfway should be added.

T (F) 6. Braising in an uncovered pan allows the item to cook without scorching.

Braising in a covered pan allows the item to cook without scorching.

(Continued)

Activity C ***(Continued)*** **Name** ______________________________

Part 2: Stewing

Circle the clue in parentheses that best completes each of the following statements.

7. Stews made by braising technique are most often prepared with (**poultry**) (**red meats**).

8. Simmering and braising cooking methods are called *stewing* when (**the cooking time is much longer**) (**the food being cooked is in bite-sizes pieces**) (**a stewing pan is used**).

9. Aromatic vegetables are often added (**at the beginning**) (**near the end**) of the cooking time.

10. Stews become rich as a result of the (**shorter cooking process required**) (**blending of flavors of the many ingredients**).

11. Vegetables other than aromatics should be (**added at the beginning of cooking time**) (**added to the stew in accordance to their cooking time**).

Notes

Fish and Shellfish Identification 34

Crossword

Chapter 34 **Name** ______________________________

Activity A **Date** ____________**Period**____________

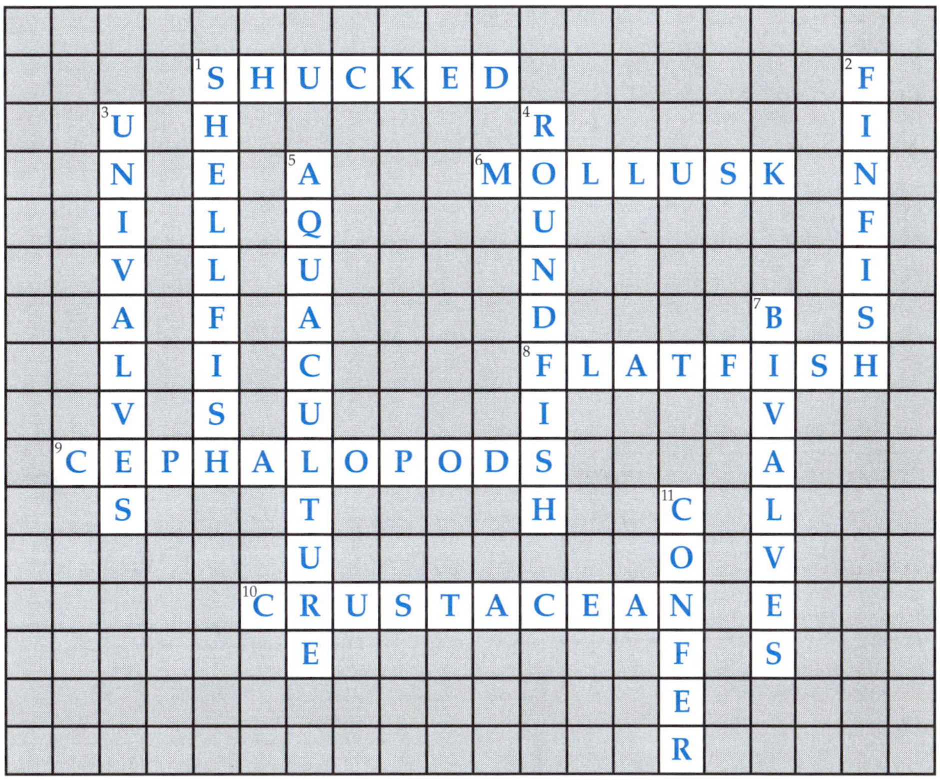

Across

1. Term that describes the process of separating the contents of a bivalve from its shell.
6. Family that consists of univalves, bivalves, and cephalopods.
8. Fish with two eyes on one side of their head and no eyes on the other side.
9. A category of mollusks known for its long arms that are covered with suckers, well-developed eyes, and sac that holds and ejects ink.
10. An aquatic species that has a hard and segmented exoskeleton, or shell.

Down

1. Water creatures that have no bones but their bodies are covered by hard external surfaces.
2. All species of fish that have an internal skeleton and swim in water.
3. Shellfish that have only one shell.
4. Fish with one eye on each side of their head and swim through the water with their dorsal fin upright. (two words)
5. The farming of fish and shellfish.
7. Shellfish that have two shells.
11. To grant.

Recognizing Fresh Fish and Shellfish

Chapter 34 Name ____________________

Activity B Date __________ Period __________

Part 1: Finfish

Complete the table below using information from the textbook.

Fish	Types	Characteristics of Flesh	Water–Fresh (F) Salt (S)
Marlin	blue, striped, black	white sometimes with pink, dense, meaty flesh	S
Catfish	farm-raised, wild	white, dense textured flesh with mild or muddy flavor	F
Tuna	bluefin, yellowfin, albacore	white to dark red, dense, chewy, moderate	S
Lake Trout	steelhead, brown	soft, orange flesh with mild flavor	F
Halibut	Atlantic, Pacific	white, moderately toothy texture, mild flavor	S
Snapper	American red, yellowtail	white, moderately flaky, sweet flavor	S
Cod	Atlantic, Pacific	white to opaque flesh with very flaky texture, mild flavor	S
Sturgeon	white	high oil content, firm textured flesh with mild flavor	F
Flounder	fluke, gray sole, blackback, rex sole	white, flaky textured flesh with mild flavor	S
Pacific Salmon	chinook, coho, pink, sockeye	pink, moderately flaky and oily, slightly strong flavor	S
Grouper	red, black	rosy-white, large flakes, firm texture, moderate flavor	S
Trout	brook, rainbow	translucent white to rose flesh, tender flake, mild flavor	F

(Continued)

Activity B ***(Continued)*** **Name** ____________________

Part 2: Shellfish

For each of the following terms or phrases, place a check (✓) in the column for the type of shellfish being described.

	Crustacean	Mollusks		
		Bivalve	Univalve	Cephalopod
Crab	✓			
Crayfish	✓			
Hard-shell clams		✓		
Has a hard, segmented shell, or exoskeleton	✓			
Has long arms covered with suckers				✓
Has one shell			✓	
Has two shells		✓		
Maine lobster	✓			
Mussels		✓		
Octopus				✓
Oysters		✓		
Rock (Spiny) lobster	✓			
Scallops		✓		
Shrimp	✓			
Soft-shell clams		✓		
Squid				✓

Judging the Quality of Fish and Shellfish

Chapter 34 Name ____________________________

Activity C Date ___________ Period ___________

Circle the clue in parentheses that best completes each of the following statements.

1. When judging the freshness of finfish, the gills should be a (**bright grey or brown**) (**bright rosy color**).
2. Fresh fish should have eyes that are (**flat and cloudy**) (**bulging and clear**) (**sunken and dry**).
3. Scales that (**are firmly attached to the skin**) (**come off easily when rubbed**) indicate a fish is fresh.
4. A fresh saltwater fish should smell (**strong and pungent**) (**ocean-like**) around the (**head and gills**) (**gut and head**) (**gills and gut**).
5. Fresh fish should feel (**firm but leave a distinct impression**) (**flabby but leave a slight impression**) (**firm and leave no impression**) when pressed.
6. Fresh cuts from saltwater fish should have a (**strong, salty smell**) (**pleasant oceanlike aroma**).
7. Boneless cuts from fresh fish should (**show no line**) (**show a clear line**) at the crease when the cut is gently folded and unfolded.
8. Both octopus and squid should have (**a distinct strong smell**) (**no particularly strong smell**).
9. Squid and octopus should be (**soft but firm**) (**hard and stiff**) (**firm and slightly elastic**).
10. Dark discoloration, especially on the body of the octopus or wings of the squid, is (**a warning sign the product may be old or has been mishandled**) (**totally normal and no indication of quality**).

Farming and Processing Fish

Chapter 34 **Name** ______________________

Activity D **Date** ____________ **Period** ____________

Part 1: Processed Fish Products

Read each statement below. Circle the letter *T* if the statement is true. If the statement is false, circle *F* and write the corrected statement on the lines that follow.

T (F) 1. It is possible to thaw individual pieces of shrimp from block frozen shrimp.

It is necessary to thaw the entire block of frozen shrimp at once.

T (F) 2. Traditionally, fish were preserved in salt because the large amount of salt drew moisture into the fish keeping it fresh and free from bacterial growth.

The large amount of salt used for preserving causes moisture to leave the fish, which makes bacterial growth impossible.

(T) F 3. Marinated herring is an example of seafood preserved in acidic liquid.

T (F) 4. Seafood to be salted is generally smoked first.

Seafood to be smoked is generally salted first.

T (F) 5. Most smoked products do not need refrigeration.

Most smoked seafood products must still be refrigerated.

T (F) 6. Canned products are raw, shelf stable, and often less expensive than the fresh equivalent.

Canned products are fully cooked, shelf stable, and often less expensive than the fresh equivalent.

(Continued)

Activity D *(Continued)* **Name** ____________________

Part 2: Aquaculture, Inspection, and Regulation

Read each statement below. Circle the letter *T* if the statement is true. If the statement is false, circle *F* and write the corrected statement on the lines that follow.

(T) F 7. Aquaculture takes place both in the wild or within man-made structures.

T (F) 8. Some of the most common aquaculture products include salmon, swordfish, and halibut.

Some of the most common aquaculture products include salmon, hybrid bass, catfish, oysters, mussels, trout, and shrimp.

T (F) 9. There is general agreement that aquaculture has a positive effect on the environment.

People have conflicting views of aquaculture.

T (F) 10. Chefs, in general, find no difference between wild and aquaculture products.

Some chefs believe that aquaculture products lack the flavor of wild fish.

(T) F 11. Inspection and grading of fish and seafood products are voluntary and provided by the National Oceanic and Atmospheric Administration (NOAA) Seafood Inspection Program.

T (F) 12. The US Department of Agricultures confers, or grants, inspection and grade marks.

The US Department of Commerce (USDC) confers, or grants, inspection and grade marks.

(T) F 13. Regulations for processing and importing of fish and fishery products are established and enforced by the US Food and Drug Administration (FDA).

Fish and Shellfish Preparation and Cookery

35

Identifying Basic Fabrication Forms of Fish

Chapter 35 **Name** ____________________

Activity A **Date** __________ **Period** __________

Part 1

Match the following terms and identifying statements.

__F__ 1. A totally edible product with no skin or bones.

__C__ 2. A fish that has its head and collar removed and its tail and fins trimmed.

__B__ 3. Fish that has been slit on the belly and its internal organs removed.

__G__ 4. Crosscut individual portions that often include the backbone and skin.

__H__ 5. The entire fish, as it was when it was caught.

__E__ 6. The muscle that has been removed from the carcass of the fish.

__A__ 7. Fish without the head, collar, or narrow tail section allowing for uniform steaks to be cut.

__D__ 8. The first part of the fish that begins to deteriorate before fabrication.

A. center cut
B. drawn
C. dressed
D. entrails
E. fillet
F. skinless fillets
G. steaks
H. whole

Part 2

Circle the clue in parentheses that best completes each of the following statements.

9. It is uncommon to buy (**center cut**) (**drawn**) (**whole**) fish.
10. Fish are sold drawn because this form (**allows oil to drain**) (**improves shelf life**).
11. A variety of the fillet fabrication form is (**butterfly**) (**round**) (**flat**).
12. The fabrication form (**center cut**) (**dressed**) (**whole**) is commonly done with trout and other small fish that will be panfried, baked, or grilled.
13. A variety of the fillet fabrication form is (**suprêmes**) (**gutted**) (**flat**).

Reviewing Key Concepts

Chapter 35 **Name** ______________________

Activity B **Date** __________ **Period** __________

Part 1: Preparing Shellfish for Cooking

Read each statement below. Circle the letter *T* if the statement is true. If the statement is false, circle *F* and write the corrected statement on the lines that follow.

(T) F 1. Sometimes the last section of the shell and tail of shrimp may be left on for presentation.

____

____

T (F) 2. The dark vein along the back of shrimp enhances the taste of the product.

The dark vein along the back of shrimp is the digestive tract and should be removed.

T (F) 3. Clams need to be debearded by pulling off the fibers that stick out of the shell.

Mussels need to be debearded by pulling off the fibers that stick out of the shell.

T (F) 4. To open an oyster, hold the oyster on the work surface with the cupped part of the shell on top.

To open an oyster, hold the oyster on the work surface with the cupped part of the shell on the bottom.

(T) F 5. Take care to leave the detached oyster whole and uncut.

____

____

(Continued)

Activity B ***(Continued)*** **Name** ____________________

Part 2: Storing and Handling Fresh Finfish and Shellfish

Read each statement below. Circle the letter *T* if the statement is true. If the statement is false, circle *F* and write the corrected statement on the lines that follow.

(T) F 6. Fresh fish must be stored on crushed ice because most commercial refrigeration is not cold enough to store it safely.

____

____

T (F) 7. When stored on ice, a way must be found to keep the melting water on the fish.

When fish is stored on ice, there must be a way for the water from the melting ice to drain away.

T (F) 8. Whole or drawn fish can be placed directly on the ice, but must be left uncovered.

Whole or drawn fish can be placed directly on the ice and must also be completely covered with additional ice.

(T) F 9. Mollusks should be stored at 40°F (4°C) to keep them alive.

____

____

T (F) 10. Cephalopods should be stored in the same manner as mollusks.

Cephalopods should be stored in the same manner as fillets.

____

Dry- and Moist-Heat Cooking

Chapter 35 **Name** ______________________________

Activity C **Date** ____________ **Period** ____________

Part 1: Dry-Heat Methods

Circle the clue in parentheses that best completes each of the following statements.

1. Many chefs prefer (**clarified butter**) (**fish oil**) (**shortening**) for sautéing fish.
2. Browned butter is a classical preparation called (**beurre noisette**) (**court bouillon**) (**pin bones**).
3. Thick pieces of fish that are not completely cooked after sautéing, may be (**sliced and recooked**) (**deep fried**) (**finished in the oven**).
4. Fish is always dredged in (**clarified butter**) (**breading or batter**) (**salt**) before panfrying.
5. Fish should be deep-fried until the coating is (**light tan**) (**golden brown**) (**dark brown**).
6. The most important consideration for grilling fish is the (**size of the grill**) (**choice of fish**).
7. (**Firm-fleshed**) (**Soft-fleshed**) fish are best for grilling.
8. Broiling is an easy way to cook (**some firm-fleshed varieties of fish**) (**only delicate shellfish**) (**most any variety of fish or seafood**).
9. For delicately textured fish and seafood items, (**broiling**) (**baking**) lessens the chance of overcooking.
10. When grilling, more (**delicate**) (**firm**) items may be finished in the oven.

Part 2: Moist-Heat Methods

Circle the clue in parentheses that best completes each of the following statements.

11. Deep poaching is best for (**large, whole dressed**) (**small, filleted**) fish.
12. The preferred liquid for deep poaching is (**beurre noisette**) (**court bouillon**) (**pin bones**).
13. The poaching method that fully covers the item is (**deep**) (**shallow**) poaching.
14. The poaching method that partially covers the item is (**deep**) (**shallow**) poaching.
15. Steaming is a cooking method best used on (**tender fish**) (**firm fish**) (**shellfish**).
16. Fish, cooked by any method, should be cooked only long enough to allow the (**protein to fully coagulate**) (**juices to run clear**) (**skin to fully brown**).

Hot Sandwiches and Pizza

36

Hot Sandwiches and Their Ingredients

Chapter 36 **Name** ____________________

Activity A **Date** __________ **Period** __________

Part 1

Read each statement below. Circle the letter *T* if the statement is true. If the statement is false, circle *F* and write the corrected statement on the lines that follow.

(T) F 1. There is little difference between hot and cold sandwiches other than part or all of a hot sandwich is served hot.

____

____

T (F) 2. Most hot sandwiches contain several hot fillings.

Many hot sandwiches contain only one or two hot fillings.

____

T (F) 3. Hot sandwiches can be divided into two categories—sandwiches made using hot fillings and those made using deep-fried ingredients.

Hot sandwiches can be divided into two categories—sandwiches made using hot fillings and whole cooked sandwiches.

T (F) 4. Hot sandwiches that mix hot and cold ingredients are best when temperatures are balanced and the whole sandwich is lukewarm.

To serve hot sandwiches successfully, the hot components must be hot and the other components must remain cool.

(T) F 5. Hamburger must be cooked to a minimum of 155°F (68°C) to ensure that any *E. coli* in the meat is dead.

____

____

(Continued)

Activity A *(Continued)* **Name** ______________________

T (F) 6. Sandwiches made from deep-fried ingredients are best prepared early and kept in a warmer.

Sandwiches made from deep-fried ingredients are best prepared at the last moment possible.

(T) F 7. Whole cooked sandwiches differ from hot filling sandwiches in that the entire sandwich is cooked and served hot.

____

____

T (F) 8. For large volume or fast-paced operations, sautéed or griddled whole cooked sandwiches should be assembled at the last possible moment.

For large volume or fast-paced operations, sautéed or griddled whole cooked sandwiches should be assembled in advance, held in the cooler until needed, and cooked when an order is received.

Part 2

Circle the clue in parentheses that best completes each of the following statements.

9. Hamburgers, chicken breasts, eggs, and pork chops are frequently served as (**deep-fried or griddled**) (**whole cooked**) (**sautéed or griddled**) ingredients for hot sandwiches.
10. Checking the finished cooked product for a meat or fish sandwich with an instant-read thermometer is (**acceptable but unnecessary**) (**a good idea**) (**essential**).
11. Steaks can be cooked to a lesser degree than hamburger meat because *E. coli* is (**located on the surface of**) (**unable to live on**) a solid piece of meat.
12. Deep-fried ingredients have the advantage of adding (**crunch**) (**concentrated heat**) (**moisture**) to a hot sandwich.
13. If it is necessary to hold deep-fried ingredients, hold them (**covered**) (**uncovered**) in a warmer.
14. Deep-fried sandwiches have a higher fat content and therefore, (**benefit from**) (**are unsuitable for**) spicy, acidic, and fresh condiments.

(Continued)

Activity A *(Continued)* **Name** ______________________________

15. Catfish, oysters, chicken breast, and falafel are some common (**griddled**) (**sautéed**) (**poached**) (**deep-fried**) sandwich ingredients.
16. Poaching is (**rarely**) (**often**) used to cook or heat hot sandwich ingredients.
17. (**Poaching**) (**Boiling**) is the best cooking method for sausages.
18. Grilled cheese sandwiches really are (**grilled**) (**sautéed or griddled**) (**toasted**).
19. A tool for cooking sandwiches that consists of two hot, smooth surfaces that close on the top and bottom of the sandwich is called a (**panini grill**) (**clamshell griddle**).
20. A tool for cooking sandwiches that consists of two hot surfaces with ridges that leave grill marks on the cooked sandwich is called a (**panini grill**) (**clamshell griddle**).
21. The most well-known example of a whole deep-fried sandwich is the (**tuna melt**) (**Monte Cristo**).
22. Whole baked sandwiches that are wrapped before cooking produce a (**more flavorful**) (**drier**) sandwich.

Making Pizza

Chapter 36 **Name** ____________________

Activity B **Date** __________ **Period** __________

Part 1

Read each statement below. Circle the letter *T* if the statement is true. If the statement is false, circle *F* and write the corrected statement on the lines that follow.

(T) F 1. Pizza is a flatbread that is cooked in a hot oven with an assortment of toppings.

T (F) 2. Pizza dough is significantly different from bread dough.

Pizza begins with yeast dough that is similar to bread dough.

T (F) 3. A pizza peel is a large spatula used to spread toppings on pizza.

A pizza peel is a long-handled, large spatula that is used to slide the pizza in and out of the oven.

(T) F 4. Thin crust pizza will have a crisp crust if it is baked directly on the oven floor or on a perforated pizza pan.

(T) F 5. Deep-dish pizza and thin crust pizza both begin with a circle of pizza dough.

T (F) 6. Deep-dish pizza is always baked directly on the oven floor in a moderate oven.

Deep-dish pizza is baked in the pan in a hot oven.

(Continued)

Activity B *(Continued)* **Name** ______________________________

Part 2

Circle the clue in parentheses that best completes each of the following statements.

7. Deep-dish pizza dough is rolled (**thicker than**) (**thinner than**) (**the same thickness as**) thin crust pizza dough is rolled.

8. Deep-dish pizza dough is rolled out several inches (**smaller**) (**larger**) than the size of the deep-dish pizza pan.

9. The cheese of choice for pizza is (**Parmesan**) (**American**) (**mozzarella**).

10. The sequence for adding toppings to pizza after the dough has been rolled out is
(**grated cheese, other toppings, then tomato sauce**)
(**tomato sauce, cheese, then other toppings**)
(**tomato sauce, other toppings, then cheese**).

11. A calzone is (**often served as an appetizer**)
(**dough that is filled, folded in half, and deep fried**)
(**dough that is filled, folded in half, and baked**).

12. Stromboli (**originated in Italy**)
(**is a large roll or stuffed bread that is baked and sliced to order**)
(**dough that is filled, folded in half, and deep fried**).

13. Panzerotti (**is often served as an appetizer**) (**originated in Philadelphia**) (**is deep fried**).

Notes

Dairy and Egg Identification 37

Terminology

Chapter 37 Name ______________________

Activity A Date ____________ Period ____________

Match the following terms and identifying statements. Terms may be used more than once.

__B__ 1. An ingredient that causes milk to thicken dramatically when making cheese.

__I__ 2. The watery portion of milk that contains one type of protein in milk.

__F__ 3. Process that permanently and evenly distributes the butterfat in milk.

__B__ 4. Rennet is an example of this type of ingredient.

__E__ 5. A term for trays that hold 30 eggs.

__A__ 6. Rapid mixing of cream that produces butter.

__H__ 7. Heating milk to 280°F (138°C) for 2 to 6 seconds.

__D__ 8. Part of milk that contains the casein proteins.

__G__ 9. The main carbohydrate in milk.

__D__ 10. This is placed in a mold and, as it ages, knits together to form cheese.

__G__ 11. Also called a sugar, although it is not sweet to taste.

__C__ 12. The removal of water to make milk a less-dilute liquid.

A. churning
B. coagulant
C. concentration
D. curds
E. flats
F. homogenization
G. lactose
H. ultra high temperature (UHT) pasteurization
I. whey

Using Technology to Alter Milk Composition

Chapter 37 **Name** ______________________

Activity B **Date** __________ **Period** __________

Part 1: Basic Composition of Milk

Complete the pictograph below by dividing the "glass of whole milk" into sections that represent the percentage of each component found in milk. Complete the callout labels and draw an arrow from each label to the corresponding section of the graph.

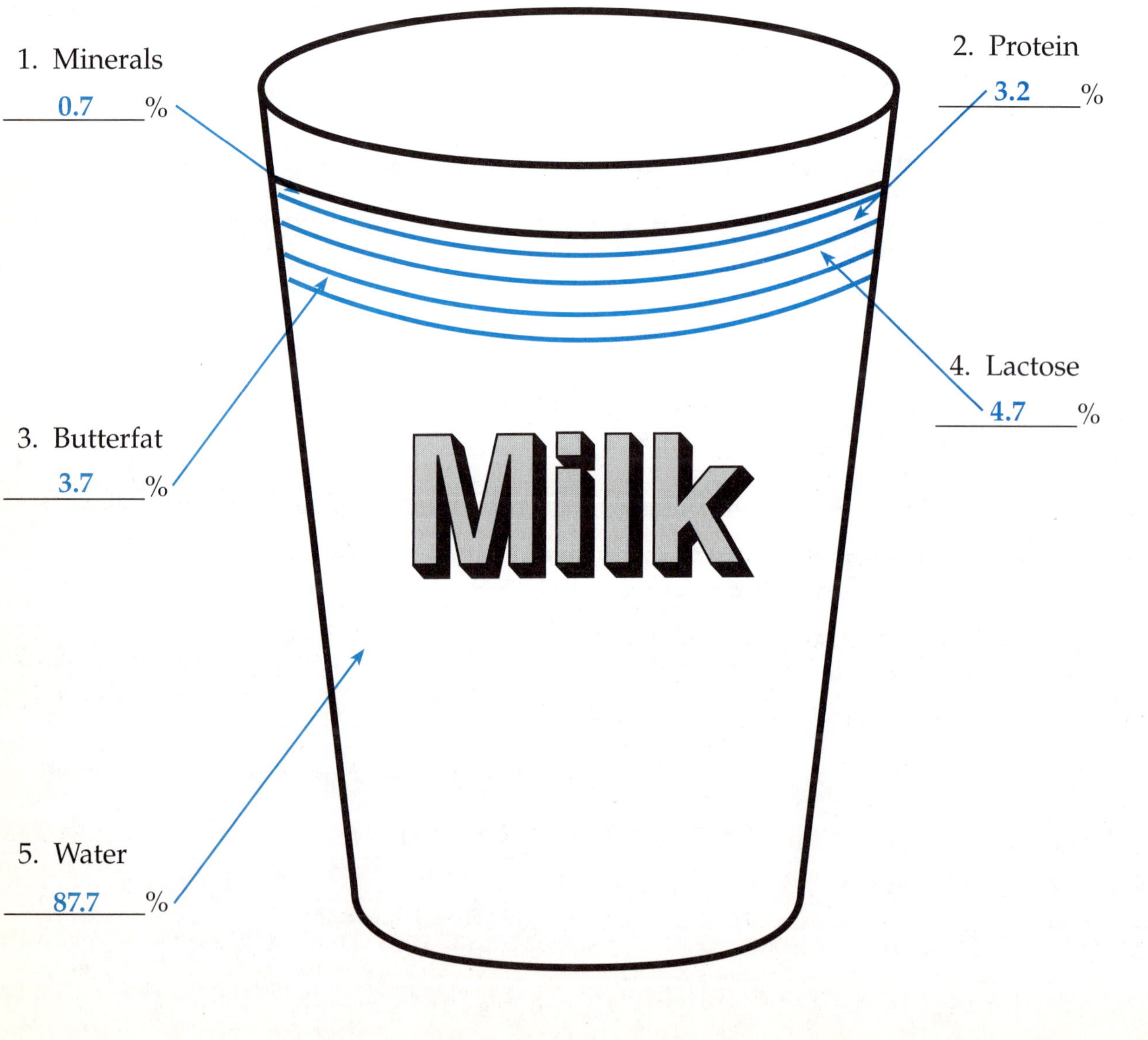
1. Minerals
0.7 %
2. Protein
3.2 %
3. Butterfat
3.7 %
4. Lactose
4.7 %
5. Water
87.7 %
Milk

(Continued)

Activity B ***(Continued)*** **Name** ______________________

Part 2: Changing Butterfat Content

Read each statement below. Circle the letter ***T*** if the statement is true. If the statement is false, circle ***F*** and write the corrected statement on the lines that follow.

(T) F 6. A centrifuge spins milk at high speeds to separate the butterfat from the rest of milk.

____

____

T (F) 7. All the butterfat is removed from milk before it is sold.

Butterfat content is adjusted.

____

(T) F 8. Both milk and high butterfat products are defined by their levels of butterfat.

____

____

T (F) 9. Removed butterfat is discarded.

The butterfat removed during centrifuging is used to create high

butterfat dairy products.

Part 3: Changing Concentration

Match the following terms and identifying statements. Answer the questions that follow.

C 10. Milk that has 60 percent of the water removed and a large amount of sugar added. A thick, rich, very sweet product that is canned and commonly used in baked products.

B 11. Milk that has 60 percent of the water removed. This thick, rich product is sold canned.

A 12. Skim milk that has nearly all of the water removed during a drying process. The resulting white powder does not require refrigeration and has a long shelf life.

A. dried milk powder

B. evaporated milk

C. sweetened condensed milk

(Continued)

Activity B *(Continued)* **Name** ______________________

13. What effect does removing water from milk have on the level of protein in the milk?

    As water is removed from the milk, the level of protein increases.

14. What effect does removing water from milk have on the level of sugar in the milk?

    As water is removed from the milk, the level of sugar increases.

15. What effect does removing water from milk have on the level of butterfat in the milk?

    As water is removed from the milk, the level of butterfat increases.

Reviewing Key Concepts

Chapter 37 **Name** ______________________________

Activity C **Date** ____________ **Period** ____________

Part 1

Circle the clue in parentheses that best completes each of the following statements.

1. Butter is made by rapid mixing or (**pasteurization**) (**churning**) (**UHT**) of cream.
2. As the cream is mixed to make butter, lumps of (**lactose**) (**curds**) (**butterfat**) emerge and begin to stick together to form larger and larger pieces of butter.
3. A purchase form of butter that is individually wrapped, one-pound pieces is typically called (**butterfats**) (**butter prints**) (**butter sticks**).
4. Grocery stores commonly sell butter in individually wrapped, quarter-pound sticks; packed (**four**) (**six**) (**eight**) to a box and (**12**) (**24**) (**36**) boxes to a case.
5. Whipped butter is butter mixed with (**curds**) (**lactose**) (**nitrogen**) to make it fluffy.
6. Cultured dairy products are the result of adding (**friendly bacteria**) (**nitrogen**) to milk.
7. The substance that thickens a cultured dairy product during the incubation period is (**lactic acid**) (**nitrogen**) (**friendly bacteria**).
8. The color of an egg shell (**is**) (**is not**) an indication of quality.
9. Within the egg white is a twisted white cord that connects the (**yolk to the white**) (**yolk to the shell**) (**white to the shell**). The cord (**is**) (**is not**) edible.
10. The egg white of a fresh egg is (**thick**) (**thin**); the white of an old egg is (**thick**) (**thin**).
11. The egg (**white**) (**yolk**) contains most of the nutrients in an egg.
12. Eggs have an air pocket between the shell and the egg white at one end. As the egg gets older the pocket gets (**smaller**) (**larger**).
13. The most common purchase forms of eggs are (**shell eggs, pasteurized eggs, blends, dried, and hard-cooked**) (**shell eggs, homogenized eggs, blends, dried, and parboiled**).
14. Eggs and dairy products (**are**) (**are not**) susceptible to spoilage.
15. Dairy and egg products must be kept (**away from light**) (**under refrigeration**).
16. Eggs and dairy products (**can**) (**cannot**) absorb flavors such as onions and garlic.
17. Eggs with a crack in the shell (**are safe**) (**are not safe**) to use.
18. Buttermilk, yogurt, and sour cream are (**homogenization**) (**cultured**) dairy products.

Activity C ***(Continued)*** **Name** ______________________

Part 2

Match the following terms and identifying statements. Some terms will be used more than once.

F	19. Have elastic or creamy texture. When well aged, they can become runny.		A. blue cheeses
G	20. Also called *pasta filata*.		B. fresh cheeses
A	21. The color of these cheeses is a type of edible mold.		C. hard cheeses
D	22. Feel firm but are still elastic, and are aged for at least a month before being sold.		D. medium firm cheeses
C	23. The driest cheeses, and therefore have a very long shelf lives.		E. processed cheeses
E	24. Begins with grated cheeses that are melted and mixed with an emulsifier, water, and sometimes additional fat.		F. soft cheeses
B	25. High moisture cheeses that are barely aged at all.		G. stretched cheeses
D	26. Examples included Morbier, Monterey Jack, Fontina, and Colby.		
A	27. Examples include Roquefort, Stilton, Gorgonzola, and Maytag Blue.		
F	28. Examples include Brie, Camembert, and lightly aged goat cheeses also known as *chevre*.		
E	29. Formed into blocks or squirted into jars.		
B	30. Spoil more easily than other cheeses.		
G	31. To make these cheeses, hot curds are repeatedly stretched.		
C	32. When these cheeses become very hard, they are referred to as grating cheeses.		
E	33. The most famous member of this family is American cheese.		
B	34. Examples include cream cheese, cottage cheese, and ricotta.		
G	35. Examples include mozzarella, string cheese, and Provolone.		
C	36. Examples include Parmesan, Cheddar, Swiss, Manchego, Gruyère, and Romano.		

Breakfast Cookery

38

Terminology

Chapter 38 **Name** ________________

Activity A **Date** ________ **Period** ________

Match the egg preparations with the descriptions of their cooking processes.

__B__ 1. The chef gently lowers two shell eggs directly into a pan of simmering water. As soon as the water returns to a simmer, the chef sets a timer to two minutes. When the timer goes off, the chef removes the eggs and places them in eggcups for service.

__F__ 2. The chef breaks three eggs into a mixing bowl and whisks in a little milk, salt, and pepper. The chef heats just enough butter in a nonstick pan to coat the bottom. When the butter begins to bubble, the chef pours in the egg mixture and stirs just until the eggs began to coagulate. Once the eggs form into a cohesive mass, the chef sprinkles cheese over the top, folds the mass over to form a half circle, and places it on the serving plate.

__A__ 3. The chef cracks two eggs directly into a pan of hot butter. As the eggs cook over moderate heat, the chef spoons the hot butter in the pan over the top of the eggs to lightly cook the yolks. The eggs are removed from the pan without flipping.

__D__ 4. The chef soaks bread slices in a mixture of egg and milk, then fries the soaked bread on a griddle. The slices are flipped over and cooked until both sides are golden brown.

__H__ 5. The chef cracks two eggs directly into a pan of hot butter. When the eggs are cooked to the desired doneness, the chef slides them out of the pan and onto a plate with the yolks facing up.

A. basted eggs

B. coddled eggs

C. eggs over

D. French toast

E. frittata

F. omelet

G. poached eggs

H. sunny-side up eggs

(Continued)

Activity A *(Continued)* **Name** ______________________

__C__ 6. The chef cracks two eggs directly into a pan of hot butter and cooks them just until the whites are fully coagulated. Then the chef carefully flips the eggs over and continues to cook them to the doneness ordered by the customer.

__E__ 7. The chef breaks three eggs into a mixing bowl and whisks in a little milk, salt, pepper, and herbs. The chef pours the egg mixture into a nonstick pan containing a small amount of hot butter. The chef stirs just until the eggs began to coagulate. When the eggs form a cohesive mass and brown, the chef flips the mass to allow the topside to brown. When top and bottom are browned, the chef slides the egg mass onto the serving plate without folding.

__G__ 8. The chef cracks an egg into a small bowl and lowers the egg carefully into gently boiling water to which some vinegar has been added. The chef uses a slotted spoon to swirl the egg to form a round shape with the white enveloping the yolk. After three minutes, the chef uses the slotted spoon to lift the egg from the water and into a serving bowl.

A. basted eggs
B. coddled eggs
C. eggs over
D. French toast
E. frittata
F. omelet
G. poached eggs
H. sunny-side up eggs

Cooking Breakfast Meats

Chapter 38 Name ______________________________

Activity B Date ___________ Period ___________

Circle the clue in parentheses that best completes each of the following statements.

1. Ham is best (**quickly**) (**slowly**) panfried or grilled to keep it moist and tender.
2. Breakfast sausage is made (**only from pork**) (**from ground pork, chicken, and turkey**) (**from beef, chicken, and pork**).
3. Sausage links (**have**) (**do not have**) casings.
4. Sausage patties (**have**) (**do not have**) casings.
5. In most commercial kitchens, bacon is cooked (**by panfrying**) (**by grilling**) (**in the oven**).
6. Breakfast sausages are (**panfried**) (**deep fried**) or grilled until done.
7. Nicely shaped strips and even cooking are two advantages of cooking bacon (**by panfrying**) (**by grilling**) (**in the oven**).
8. Regardless of how crisp the final product will be, bacon should be cooked until (**the red is very dark**) (**the strip is no longer shiny**) (**no white fat is visible**).
9. Professional kitchens often prepare breakfast sausage (**by deep frying**) (**by broiling**) (**by baking it in the oven**).
10. Canadian bacon is (**thick bacon**) (**thin ham**) (**boneless pork loin**).
11. Canadian bacon is cooked the same as (**bacon**) (**ham**).
12. Breakfast sausages should be cooked (**rare**) (**medium**) (**well-done**).
13. Many commercial kitchens purchase bacon that is already (**cut into bite-sized lengths**) (**laid out on ovenproof parchment paper**) (**separated into serving size portions**).
14. Professional cooks frequently cook ham (**by broiling**) (**by steaming**) (**in the oven**).

Reviewing Key Concepts

Chapter 38 Name ______________________

Activity C Date __________ Period __________

Part 1: Breakfast Batters

Read each statement below. Circle the letter *T* if the statement is true. If the statement is false, circle *F* and write the corrected statement on the lines that follow.

T (F) 1. The batter for French toast is a mixture of eggs, milk, and fat.

French toast is made from bread soaked in a milk and egg mixture.

T (F) 2. Pancakes are a form of quick bread that is baked in the oven.

Pancakes are a form of quick bread that is cooked in a pan or griddle.

T (F) 3. Pancakes are leavened with yeast.

Pancakes are leavened with baking soda or baking powder.

(T) F 4. Overmixing pancake batter can result in dense or tough pancakes.

T (F) 5. Turn pancakes when bubbles appear on the surface and the bottom is still white.

Turn the pancakes when bubbles appear on the surface and the bottom is golden brown.

(T) F 6. Pancakes must be served as soon as possible, because they may become dry and flat if held over a period of time.

(Continued)

Activity C ***(Continued)*** **Name** ____________________

T (F) 7. Waffles are a quick bread that has a batter that is a little thinner and contains less fat than pancake batter.

Waffles are a quick bread like pancakes, but the batter is thicker and contains more fat.

(T) F 8. The batter for French toast can be varied by adding different flavorings to the batter.

T (F) 9. To assure that waffles are crisp and don't stick, start waffle in a cold waffle iron.

To assure that waffles are crisp and don't stick, start waffle in a preheated waffle iron.

Part 2: Hot Cereals

Read each statement below. Circle the letter *T* if the statement is true. If the statement is false, circle *F* and write the corrected statement on the lines that follow.

T (F) 10. The proper ratio of liquid to cereal and the amount of time needed for cooking is essentially the same for all types of cereal grains.

The ratio of liquid to cereal and the cooking time vary depending on the type of grain and how it was processed.

T (F) 11. Cereal should be cooked until it is dry.

Cook the cereal until it is smooth and moist, with no lumps.

T (F) 12. Once placed in a steam table, the consistency of hot cereal will hold for hours.

Hot cereals continue to thicken when held in a steam table.

T (F) 13. Hot cereals are a nutritious source of B vitamins and fat.

Hot cereals are a nutritious source of B vitamins and fiber.

(Continued)

Activity C *(Continued)* **Name** ______________________

T (F) 14. Farina is a cereal made from processed rice.

Farina is a cereal made from processed and ground wheat.

T (F) 15. Grits is a cereal made from ground wheat.

Grits is a cereal made from coarsely ground hominy corn.

T (F) 16. Steel cut oatmeal has a finer texture and requires less cooking time than rolled oats.

Steel cut oatmeal has a coarse texture and requires a longer cooking time.

(T) F 17. Rice cereals that are cracked are typically cooked to a smooth consistency.

Food Presentation

39

Terminology

Chapter 39 Name ______________________

Activity A Date __________ Period __________

Match the following terms and identifying statements. Terms may be used more than once.

Answer	Statement
F	1. A balanced arrangement that is identical on opposite sides of a center point.
D	2. The location or item to which the eye is first drawn when looking at a plate presentation.
B	3. A decorative covered stand that keeps food hot.
E	4. Edible decorative addition or accompaniment to a dish.
A	5. A sense of balance achieved by artistically arranging items without creating two identical sides of a center point.
B	6. Enables chefs to serve hot foods at optimal temperatures at a buffet presentation.
E	7. Should improve appearance but never detract from the main dish.
D	8. Usually the highest, biggest, or most colorful item on the plate.
C	9. Neglect of any plating principles can diminish an otherwise successful presentation.

A. asymmetry
B. chafing dish
C. detract
D. focal point
E. garnish
F. symmetry

Applying Presentation Principles

Chapter 39 Name ____________________

Activity B Date __________ Period __________

Part 1: Plating

Circle the clue in parentheses that best completes each of the following statements.

1. When planning plate presentation, foods that have (**similar**) (**contrasting**) vibrant colors look the most appetizing.
2. The plating process should happen rapidly to protect food (**balance**) (**temperature**).
3. Proportion refers to the relationship between the (**amounts**) (**textures**) (**colors**) of the different food items on a plate.
4. When planning a plate, chefs consider how the food (**covers the plate**) (**rises above the plate**) (**covers and rises above the plate**).
5. The focal point of a plate is usually (**the main item**) (**anything red**).
6. Repeating the same shapes on the plate should be (**a goal**) (**avoided**).
7. Overly tall food is likely to appear (**formal**) (**comical**).
8. Plate designs with a definite (**predominant color**) (**focal point**) create a satisfying sense of order.
9. Properly cooked foods usually (**have**) (**do not have**) naturally vibrant colors.
10. For balance, foods on a plate should have (**similar**) (**various**) textures.
11. (**Asymmetry**) (**Proportion**) (**Symmetry**) refers to the relationship between the size of the actual plate and the food arranged on it.
12. A plate cover is a device that helps chefs apply the (**focal point**) (**variety**) (**temperature**) plating principle.
13. Topping a mound of applesauce with a thin wedge of crisp fresh apple is an example of applying the plating principle of (**height**) (**color**) (**variety of texture**).
14. Serving a cold salad in a lukewarm bowl is an example of (**balancing temperature**) (**ignoring the plating principle of temperature**).
15. Color adds to a dish and a garnish may be used to improve the color of a plate (**regardless of its taste**) (**only if its taste complements the flavors of the dish**).

(Continued)

Activity B *(Continued)* **Name** ______________________________

Part 2: Platters and Buffets

Read each statement below. Circle the letter *T* if the statement is true. If the statement is false, circle *F* and write the corrected statement on the lines that follow.

(T) F 16. On a platter, the focal point is often a centerpiece that is not meant to be eaten.

____

____

T (F) 17. Platters with too much negative space appear crowded, those with too little appear empty.

Platters with too little negative space appear crowded, those with too much appear empty.

T (F) 18. A platter with identical sides split by a center point is an example of asymmetry.

A platter with identical sides split by a center point is an example of symmetry.

T (F) 19. If the food is to be served by a cook or server, portion sizes on a platter don't matter.

The size and shape of the portions should be easy to handle whether customers are serving themselves or being served by a cook or server.

(T) F 20. The same considerations that pertain to a platter pertain to an entire buffet.

____

____

T (F) 21. Buffets are always arranged symmetrically.

Buffets can be arranged either symmetrically or asymmetrically.

____

(T) F 22. Two aspects of functionality related to buffet design to consider are keeping the buffet clean and well stocked.

____

____

(Continued)

Activity B ***(Continued)*** **Name** ______________________

T (F) 23. Buffet centerpieces are similar to platter centerpieces but generally smaller.

Buffet centerpieces are similar to platter centerpieces but generally larger.

T (F) 24. Chafing dishes are often used in buffets to keep cold foods cold.

Chafing dishes are often used in buffets to keep hot foods hot.

Garnishing Techniques

Chapter 39 **Name** ______________________________

Activity C **Date** ____________ **Period** ____________

Part 1

Circle the clue in parentheses that best completes each of the following statements.

1. Garnishes should (**coordinate**) (**contrast**) with the flavors and temperature of the dish.
2. Garnishes (**may**) (**should not**) overshadow the main dish.
3. Garnishes should be used sparingly and (**only when functional**) (**even if only for visual stimulus**).
4. Herbs suitable for garnishing hot foods include (**cilantro, chervil, and basil**) (**thyme, rosemary, and parsley**).
5. When making a scallion flower, make as many (**horizontal**) (**lengthwise**) cuts down the scallion as possible. Roll the scallion (**45°**) (**90°**) and cut a new series of slices. Place the scallion in (**hot**) (**warm**) (**cool**) (**ice**) water for at least 30 minutes.
6. When making a radish rose, begin cutting when the radish is (**cold**) (**at room temperature**). Start at the (**top**) (**bottom**) of the radish, and cut petals on the sides of the radish. Petals should be about (**1/16-inch**) (**1/8-inch**) (**1/4-inch**) thick.
7. When making a tomato rose, you create the petals of the rose from a strip of the tomato (**pulp**) (**skin**). When formed, tomato roses should be stored in (**cold water**) (**the refrigerator**). Make tomato roses (**as far ahead**) (**as close to service**) as possible.
8. When making a vegetable cutouts, begin with a (**well chilled**) (**room temperature**) vegetable. Vegetables such as (**beets, turnips, and carrots**) (**beans, squash, and white potatoes**) work well.

(Continued)

Activity C (*Continued*) **Name** ______________________

Part 2

Answer the following in the space provided.

9. List four examples of crispy garnishes.

(Answers will vary, but may include:) sliced croutons, deep-fried root vegetables, baked or deep-friend wonton wrappers, deep-fried raviolis, baked flatbreads or crackers, fleurons, cookies and sugar for pastry presentations.

10. In addition to contributing a crunch to the eating experience, crispy items add height and a sense of sculpture to the plate.

11. What are two examples of improper garnishes?

(Answers will vary, but may include:) deep-fried tortilla chips on German cuisine, lettuce on a hot appetizer, raw carrot flowers on beef stew.

Introduction to the Bakeshop

40

Terminology

Chapter 40 **Name** ______________________

Activity A **Date** __________ **Period** __________

Match the following terms and identifying statements. Not all terms will be used.

__I__ 1. The head of the baking and pastry department.

__F__ 2. The process in which yeast, in a warm moist environment, feeds on carbohydrates and gives off carbon dioxide and alcohol.

__L__ 3. The term often used to refer to fats used in the bakeshop.

__A__ 4. Food professional who prepares and bakes breads.

__C__ 5. An alkaline powder, also known as *sodium bicarbonate,* used as a chemical leavener.

__H__ 6. A process in which gases are trapped in dough creating small bubbles that give baked goods a light and airy texture.

__M__ 7. A mixture of equal parts of water and sugar by weight that is brought to a boil and simmered just until the sugar dissolves in the water.

__B__ 8. A chemical leavener that is sodium bicarbonate premixed with an acid chemical, such as cream of tartar.

__G__ 9. A rubbery substance that is responsible for giving baked goods structure.

__J__ 10. Food professional responsible for preparing sweet dessert items.

__E__ 11. Alcohol-based flavorings.

__D__ 12. Softening gelatin in cold water.

A. baker
B. baking powder
C. baking soda
D. blooming
E. extracts
F. fermentation
G. gluten
H. leavening
I. pastry chef
J. pastry cook
K. potential
L. shortening
M. simple syrup

The Chemistry of Baking

Chapter 40 **Name** ______________________

Activity B **Date** __________**Period**__________

Circle the clue in parentheses that best completes each of the following statements.

1. The main difference between the various types of flour used in the bakeshop is the (**sugar**) (**protein**) content of the flours.
2. When flour is mixed with water, the (**sugar**) (**protein**) in the flour produces gluten.
3. In professional bakeshops, wheat flours are categorized by their (**sugar**) (**gluten**) potential.
4. In addition to adding a sweet taste, sugar helps maintain (**gluten**) (**moistness**) in cakes.
5. Sugar assists in the (**mixing**) (**leavening**) process in breads.
6. Sugar is used to make cookies (**soft**) (**crisp**).
7. Fat (**lengthens**) (**shortens**) strands of gluten in dough, making the product (**less**) (**more**) tender and (**more**) (**less**) elastic or chewy.
8. Shortenings add flavor, color, richness, and (**moisture**) (**density**) to baked goods.
9. The decision of which shortening to use for a given application is based on its (**oiliness**) (**melting point**) and nutritional content.
10. Baking soda is an (**acidic**) (**alkaline**) powder used as a (**chemical**) (**yeast**) leavening agent.
11. Baking powder is (**flour**) (**baking soda**) premixed with an (**acid**) (**alkaline**) chemical.
12. Milk, buttermilk, cocoa, molasses, and cream of tartar are ingredients that can provide the (**acid**) (**alkaline**) needed for (**baking soda**) (**baking powder**) to release carbon dioxide gas.
13. Yeast is a (**chemical**) (**living microscopic plant**) (**living microscopic animal**) used to leaven bread and some baked goods.
14. (**Compressed yeast**) (**Dry yeast**) is a fresh product with a limited shelf life and should be refrigerated.

(Continued)

Activity B *(Continued)* **Name** ____________________

15. The quality of chocolate products is measured by their **(flavor, smell, appearance, texture, and melting point)** **(flavor, texture, and melting point)** **(flavor, appearance, texture, and graininess)**.

16. Chocolate liquor is composed of cocoa solids and fat called **(cocoa liquor)** **(cocoa beans)** **(cocoa butter)**.

17. When stored in conditions of fluctuating temperature or humidity, chocolate can develop a **(black)** **(white)** **(blue)** film on its surface. For this reason **(always)** **(never)** store chocolate in the refrigerator.

18. Most pastry chefs prefer **(powdered)** **(sheet)** gelatin because it is easier to use.

19. Gelatin is used to **(sweeten)** **(thicken)** **(smooth)** various sweet and savory preparations.

20. The first step in using gelatin is called **(blooming)** **(melting)** **(coloring)**, which means to soften gelatin in cold water.

21. Softened gelatin is melted or dissolved in a small amount of cold **(fat)** **(liquid)** **(leavening)**.

22. To soften powdered gelatin, mix with about **(two)** **(four)** **(six)** times its weight in cold water.

23. Store nuts in tightly sealed containers in a **(warm)** **(cool)** dark place.

24. Generally, the larger the nut pieces, the **(less)** **(more)** expensive they are.

25. Nuts **(can)** **(cannot)** be frozen for long term storage.

26. Seeds are rich in **(sugar)** **(fat)**.

27. Seeds develop a **(richer)** **(flatter)** flavor when toasted.

28. Alcohol-based flavorings are called **(pastes)** **(extracts)**.

29. Flavorings and extracts have **(mild)** **(strong)** flavors.

30. Artificial vanilla is made from a synthetic compound called **(vanilla bean)** **(vanillin)**.

Reviewing Key Concepts

Chapter 40 **Name** ______________________________

Activity C **Date** ____________ **Period** ____________

Part 1: Smallwares and Hand Tools

Match the following terms and identifying statements.

D 1. Rectangular pans used for baking bread.

F 2. Knives with thin flexible blades of various lengths and widths. They are used for spreading frostings and also as spatulas to pick up or turn items.

H 3. A piece of metal or plastic with a zigzag edge that is dragged through pastry coating or frosting to give it a decorative texture.

L 4. Shallow round pans often with fluted sides; most with removable bottoms.

A 5. A large, long-handled paddle used to slide baked goods in and out of deep ovens.

G 6. Cone-shaped bag made of cloth or plastic that has a small opening at the point of the cone into which a metal tip is placed. The bag is filled with product that is squeezed through the tip to create a decorative effect.

J 7. Also referred to as *baking sheets*. The sides are sometimes extended by using a 3-inch-high frame.

B 8. Two platforms, an ingredient scoop, and a counterweight to balance the scoop.

I 9. A single piece, either cylindrical or thin with tapered ends, that is used to roll pieces of dough into thin sheets.

M 10. Device that allows pastry cooks to frost a cake by holding a palette knife loaded with frosting stationary alongside the cake and while spinning the cake.

C 11. Round pans with straight sides used for baking cakes.

K 12. Deep cake pans with sides made of a flexible band of metal that can be opened up. These pans are used for cakes and pastries that might be hard to remove from a standard cake pan.

E 13. Sets of small round pans pressed into a single sheet of metal. Used for cupcakes or muffins.

A. baker's peel
B. balance scale
C. cake pans
D. loaf pans
E. muffin pans
F. palette knife
G. pastry bag
H. pastry comb
I. rolling pin
J. sheet pans
K. spring form pans
L. tart pans
M. turntable

(Continued)

Activity C ***(Continued)*** **Name** ______________________

Part 2: Large Equipment

Match the following terms and identifying statements.

__G__ 14. Sometimes called *roll-in ovens*, are large enough to hold an entire sheet pan rack. The rack is loaded with items to be baked and then rolled into the oven. The products are baked on the rack.

__A__ 15. An oven with a deep, wide cavity with a height of about 10 inches. Each oven is capable of holding several sheet pans. Heat can be controlled from the bottom, top, and sides for different baking effects.

__E__ 16. The three basic attachments for this appliance are the whip, paddle, and dough hook.

__F__ 17. A cabinet that will hold dough products at a warm temperature so they will rise.

__C__ 18. A mechanized rolling pin. The thickness of the rollers can be adjusted.

__H__ 19. These ovens have a series of trays set up in a Ferris wheel-like arrangement. As items are baking, the trays revolve inside the oven to allow all of the items to bake evenly.

__D__ 20. Essentially a refrigerated drum with a blade or paddle that spins inside it. Slowly turns liquid mixture into a frozen solid.

__B__ 21. A press that evenly divides a preweighed amount of dough into many smaller portions for rolls or buns.

A. deck ovens
B. dough divider
C. dough sheeter
D. ice-cream machines
E. mixers
F. proofers
G. rack ovens
H. revolving ovens

Notes

Quick Breads and Batters

41

Terminology

Chapter 41 **Name** ______________________________

Activity A **Date** ____________ **Period** ____________

Match the following terms and identifying statements. Terms may be used more than once.

__B__ 1. During the last step of this process, gluten develops and the leavening agent reacts.

__F__ 2. Individual fried pastry.

__G__ 3. The paste or thick batter used to make cream puffs and éclairs.

__B__ 4. Combines dry ingredients first; then solid shortening is cut in, and finally, liquid ingredients are added and mixed just enough to combine with the other ingredients.

__D__ 5. A mixture of flour and other ingredients that is stiff enough to form into shapes for baking.

__F, H__ 6. May be formed from a dough or from a batter.

__C__ 7. A very thin pancake.

__A__ 8. A mixture of flour and enough liquid so that the mixture is pourable.

__G__ 9. Is one of the few pastry preparations made on the stovetop.

__H__ 10. Chemically leavened baked product.

__A__ 11. Muffins, pancakes, waffles, and cream puffs all begin as this.

__C__ 12. Requires no leavening agent because it is paper-thin.

__E__ 13. To speed up.

__H__ 14. One characteristic this type of product has is soft texture; many contain a good amount of shortening, which helps create a tender product.

A. batter
B. biscuit method
C. crêpe
D. dough
E. expedite
F. fritter
G. pâte à choux
H. quick bread

The Basics of Quick Breads and Batters

Chapter 41 Name ______________________________

Activity B Date ____________ Period ____________

Circle the clue in parentheses that best completes each of the following statements.

1. Quick breads are leavened with chemical leaveners such as baking powder or baking soda; both of which act (**more quickly**) (**more slowly**) than yeast.
2. Quick breads begin in the form of (**dough**) (**batter**) (**either dough or batter**).
3. Quality quick breads are (**dense and chewy**) (**dry and flaky**) (**light and tender**).
4. Quick bread dough is often (**high**) (**low**) in moisture.
5. One ingredient used in quick bread recipes that contributes to its delicate texture is (**low**) (**balanced**) (**high**) gluten flour.
6. One ingredient used in quick bread recipes that contributes to its delicate texture is the (**limited**) (**good**) amount of shortening.
7. The manner in which the dough is prepared (**is very important**) (**is not really important**) in trying to achieve a tender texture.
8. The proportion of liquid to flour in a batter is (**the same as**) (**greater than**) (**less than**) the proportion of liquid to flour in dough.
9. Mixing (**develops**) (**hinders**) gluten in the flour of a dough.
10. Overmixing results in (**too little**) (**too much**) gluten; making the finished product (**dense and chewy**) (**dry and flaky**) (**light and tender**).
11. Most quick breads are mixed (**until all ingredients are well combined and smooth**) (**only to the point necessary to combine ingredients**).
12. Holes or tunnels inside products or poorly shaped products are likely the result of (**undermixing**) (**overmixing**).

Reviewing Key Concepts

Chapter 41 Name ______________________

Activity C Date __________ Period __________

Part 1: Types of Quick Breads

Match the following terms and identifying statements.

A 1. A savory quick bread that can be served at any meal. Some bakers demand special low-gluten, high-starch content flours made from soft wheat to ensure a light flaky product.

C 2. Small, individual fried pastries.

E 3. A quick bread popular throughout Great Britain that is leavened with baking powder or baking soda and commonly cut into a triangle shape before baking.

D 4. Individual pastries similar to cupcakes.

B 5. Is essentially a form of another quick bread but uses cornmeal as the main ingredient.

A. biscuits
B. cornbread
C. fritters
D. muffins
E. scones

Part 2: Techniques for Preparing Quick Breads

Circle the clue in parentheses that best completes each of the following statements.

6. The method for mixing biscuit dough is fairly consistent. It calls for **(adding liquid ingredients to dry ingredients, then cutting in shortening) (combining dry ingredients, cutting in shortening, then adding liquid ingredients) (adding shortening to liquid ingredients, then combining with dry ingredients)**.

7. Biscuit dough can be portioned into individual biscuits by **(using a scoop to form clumps of dough) (rolling the dough and cutting it into individual rounds) (scooping or rolling and cutting)**.

8. Biscuits should be placed on **(greased) (ungreased)** sheet pans to bake.

9. When preparing muffins, **(add liquid ingredients to dry ingredients and then cut in shortening) (combine dry ingredients, cut in shortening, and then add liquid ingredients) (add shortening to liquid ingredients and then add that mixture to dry ingredients)** and mix to combine.

10. Fritters are formed from dough that is **(yeast raised) (a quick bread) (yeast raised or quick bread)**.

11. Fritters are **(fried) (baked) (cooked on a griddle)**.

(Continued)

Activity C *(Continued)* **Name** ___________________________

Part 3: Other Products That Begin as Batters

Circle the clue in parentheses that best completes each of the following statements.

12. The paste or thick batter used to make cream puffs and éclairs is (**crêpes**) (**pâte à choux**).

13. Chefs need to add no leavening to (**crêpes**) (**pâte à choux**) (**crêpes nor pâte à choux**).

14. Crêpes are made (**with**) (**without**) (**with or without**) sugar.

15. The following technique is for making (**crêpes**) (**pâte à choux**) (**crêpes or pâte à choux**) batter: First combine the liquid, fat, sugar, and salt in a saucepot and bring to a boil. Add all the flour at once and stir immediately. Cook over moderate heat while stirring until the batter forms a ball and pulls away from the sides of the pot.

16. The following technique is for making (**crêpes**) (**pâte à choux**) (**crêpes or pâte à choux**) batter: Combine the dry ingredients, beat in the eggs, add liquid gradually. Strain to remove any lumps.

17. (**Crêpes**) (**Pâte à choux**) are cooked in a pan.

18. Eggs are added one at a time when preparing (**crêpes**) (**pâte à choux**).

19. Steam helps to leaven (**crêpes**) (**pâte à choux**).

20. Products made from batters for (**crêpes**) (**pâte à choux**) (**crêpes and pâte à choux**) can be filled with either sweet or savory fillings.

Cookies

42

Cookie Conversations

Chapter 42 | **Name** ______________________

Activity A | **Date** __________ **Period** __________

Fragments of conversation that might be overheard in a professional kitchen are listed in the left column of the chart below. Place a check (✓) in column that corresponds with the classification of cookie being discussed.

	Classification of Cookie					
	Bar	**Drop**	**Icebox**	**Rolled**	**Sheet**	**Spritz**
"The production sheet says to make 12 dozen each checkerboard and pinwheel cookies for the catered event today."			✓			
"We need to standardize the new recipe for multilayered cookies with dates, nuts, and jam."					✓	
"Please get out the large- and medium-sized rosette disks."						✓
"Portion the dough into one-pound batches and form it into a log about the length of this sheet pan."	✓					
"After you frost these brownies, cut them into 2-inch squares."					✓	
"Now shape the dough into a triangle, wrap it in plastic wrap and put it in the refrigerator to chill."			✓			
"Use the #16 portion scoop so that all of the mounds will be the same size, and be sure to leave room for the cookies to flatten out as they bake."		✓				
"These cookies are sliced and ready for their second baking."	✓					
"Roll the dough a little thinner before you cut it into shapes."				✓		
"Use the pastry bag to prepare the star-shaped cookies for the catering."						✓
"We need four dozen chocolate chip cookies and two dozen oatmeal."		✓				
"Please prepare two pounds of buttercream icing for these sugar cookies."				✓		

Reviewing Key Concepts

Chapter 42 **Name** ____________________

Activity B **Date** __________ **Period** __________

Part 1: Characteristics of a Quality Cookie

Circle the clue in parentheses that best completes each of the following statements.

1. The flavor of cookies is mostly determined by the (**baking time**) (**quality of the ingredients**) (**decorating techniques**).
2. The texture of cookies is mostly determined by (**baking time**) (**ingredients**) (**decorating techniques**).
3. Baking (**at the proper temperature and for the proper time**) (**at the proper temperature**) (**for the proper time**) is essential for proper color of cookies.
4. Choosing (**high-gluten**) (**low-gluten**) flour can make cookies tough.
5. Flavor of cookies (**is**) (**is not**) affected by how fresh the ingredients are.
6. A uniform shape (**is**) (**is not**) key to the appearance of quality cookies.
7. The more sugar added to the dough, the (**less crisp**) (**more crisp**) the cookies will be.
8. To ensure good appearance, remove cookies from the sheet as soon as they (**come out of the oven**) (**have had a chance to firm up**).
9. Careful measurement of ingredients (**is**) (**is not**) essential to achieve good cookie flavor.
10. Spending extra time mixing cookie dough causes (**more**) (**less**) gluten to develop; making the finished product (**tough**) (**light and tender**).
11. Decorating cookies uniformly is important to creating attractive cookies because (**finished cookies will taste alike**) (**cookies are often displayed in batches**).
12. Proper proportions of dough ingredients (**are**) (**are not**) necessary to achieve a pleasing flavor of quality cookies.

Part 2: Common Methods of Mixing Cookie Dough

Read each statement below. Circle the letter *T* if the statement is true. If the statement is false, circle *F* and write the corrected statement on the lines that follow.

T F 13. The creaming method is the simplest way to make cookie dough.

The one-stage method is the simplest way to make cookie dough.

____

(Continued)

Activity B *(Continued)* **Name** ______________________

T (F) 14. The first step in the creaming method is to put all the ingredients into a bowl.

The first step in the creaming method is to put the butter or

shortening, sugar, and spices into a bowl.

(T) F 15. Both the one-stage method and the creaming method are done with an electric mixer using the paddle attachment.

____

____

T (F) 16. Allow five to six minutes at moderate speed to fully blend all ingredients in the one-stage method.

Allow two to three minutes at moderate speed to fully blend all ingredients

in the one-stage method.

T (F) 17. In the creaming method, butter is mixed with sugar just until moist.

In the creaming method, butter is mixed with the sugar and spices

until smooth.

(T) F 18. One advantage of the creaming method is that it is less likely to overdevelop gluten.

____

____

T (F) 19. One advantage of the one-stage method is that it is less likely to overdevelop gluten.

A risk of the one-stage method is that it is more likely to overdevelop gluten.

____

T (F) 20. In the creaming method ingredients are mixed in the following sequence: butter is mixed with sugar; spices and liquids are added next; flour is added third; and eggs are dropped in one at a time, last.

In the creaming method ingredients are mixed in the following sequence:

butter is mixed with sugar and spices; eggs and liquids are added next; and

flour is added last.

Common Methods for Forming Cookies

Chapter 42 **Name** ____________________

Activity C **Date** __________ **Period** __________

Cookies are often classified by the method used to form the dough into a cookie. On the space provided before each of the descriptions below, write ***bar, drop, icebox, rolled, sheet,*** or ***spritz*** to indicate the method used to form the cookies.

rolled 1. Dough is rolled into a thin sheet and various shaped cutters are used to cut out the cookies. The cookie shapes are placed on a sheet pan and baked.

drop 2. A scoop is used to portion dough that is placed onto a sheet pan with enough space between for the cookies to spread during cooking.

bar 3. Cookie dough is portioned into approximately one-pound (454 g) batches and formed into logs about the length of a sheet pan. Each log is flattened and baked. When it is cooked, and still warm, the logs are sliced into one-inch (2-cm) segments to form cookies, which are baked a second time to create a hard texture.

sheet 4. Cookie batter or dough is evenly spread onto a sheet pan and baked. Later the sheet is cut into individual cookies.

icebox 5. Cookie dough is formed into a log, triangle, or other shape and then wrapped in plastic wrap or parchment paper and refrigerated. When the dough is fully chilled, it is sliced into individual cookies and baked.

spritz 6. Soft cookie dough is forced through a pastry bag to form individual shapes such as rosettes, shells, and scrolls or the dough is pressed through a specially shaped die on a cookie press.

Yeast-Raised Products

43

Terminology

Chapter 43

Activity A

Name ______________________

Date __________ **Period** __________

Match the following terms and identifying statements. Terms may be used more than once.

F 1. Step in the process that comes after the dough has risen the first time.

G 2. Portioning dough by weight.

D 3. Repeatedly folding and pressing the dough after it is mixed.

B 4. The act of cutting small slashes in the surface of risen dough.

E 5. The process in which yeast dough is allowed to rise after it is shaped and before it is baked.

C 6. The process by which carbohydrates are consumed by yeast, and alcohol and carbon dioxide are released.

D 7. The part of yeast product preparation that is done to develop gluten.

B 8. This process allows gases to escape during the baking process and also create a decorative pattern on the surface of the finished loaf.

H 9. A coating with a liquid such as beaten eggs, milk, or water.

E 10. This process can happen by placing unbaked bread in a special box or by covering it with a cloth and placing it in a warm place.

A 11. The baker's occupation.

F 12. The name of this step is not to be taken literally.

A. craft

B. docking

C. fermentation

D. kneading

E. proofing

F. punching

G. scaling

H. wash

The Science of Yeast-Raised Products

Chapter 43 **Name** ______________________

Activity B **Date** ___________ **Period** ___________

Part 1: Temperature

Circle the clue in parentheses that best completes each of the following statements.

1. Dissolving yeast in liquids at temperatures over 138°F (59°C) is not recommended because the yeast (**will still work but much more slowly**) (**could be killed and not work at all**).
2. Bakers create proper conditions for fermentation by adjusting the temperature of the (**room**) (**flour**) (**liquid**).
3. Fermentation is best done in a (**cool**) (**warm**) (**hot**) place with no drafts.
4. The temperature in a proof box is typically around (**78°F to 82°F [26°C to 28°C]**) (**100°F [38°C]**) (**138°F [59C°]**).
5. Breads are baked at varying temperatures and various times depending on their size and (**the amount of gluten in the flour**) (**the desired crispness of the finished product**).
6. Refrigeration causes baked bread to (**remain fresh longer**) (**become stale more quickly**).

Part 2: Gluten

7. Gluten is the (**carbohydrate**) (**fat**) (**protein**) that gives dough its structure and elasticity.
8. The more dough is kneaded; the (**more**) (**less**) gluten is developed.
9. How long and at what speed dough is kneaded affects gluten development which, in turn, affects the (**crispness**) (**sweetness**) (**texture**) of the finished product.

Part 3: Fermentation

10. Fermentation can take as long as (**one and a half hours**) (**two and a half hours**) (**three and a half hours**).
11. When fermentation is complete, the dough is punched to (**stop the gluten**) (**release carbon dioxide gas**) (**reactivate the yeast**).

Part 4: Proofing

12. The steam or humidity in the proof box prevents a dry crust from forming on the dough, which would (**keep it from rising**) (**allow it to over rise**).
13. Washing proofed bread with beaten egg will produce a (**pale yellow, bright**) (**golden, dull**) (**deep brown, glossy**) finish to the crust.

Reviewing Key Concepts

Chapter 43 Name ______________________

Activity C Date __________ Period __________

Part 1: Preparing the Dough

Letter the steps for preparing dough for yeast-raised products below in sequential order. The first step should be labeled *A*.

E 1. Allow the dough to ferment.

J 2. Bake.

A 3. Weigh ingredients.

B 4. Dissolve yeast in liquid.

D 5. Knead the dough.

C 6. Mix in dry ingredients.

I 7. Proof the dough.

F 8. Punch the dough.

G 9. Scale the dough.

H 10. Shape the dough.

Part 2: Shaping Yeast Breads

Indicate whether each of the classic shapes for yeast-raised products listed below is a loaf or a roll by circling the correct term.

Classic Dough Shapes					
Shape	**(Circle one)**		**Shape**	**(Circle one)**	
Bagel	(loaf)	(roll) ◯	**Knot, figure eight**	(loaf)	(roll) ◯
Baguette	(loaf) ◯	(roll)	**Knot, single**	(loaf)	(roll) ◯
Boule	(loaf) ◯	(roll)	**Pan**	(loaf) ◯	(roll)
Cloverleaf	(loaf)	(roll) ◯	**Pullman**	(loaf) ◯	(roll)
Club	(loaf)	(roll) ◯	**Ring**	(loaf)	(roll) ◯
Crescent	(loaf)	(roll) ◯	**Round**	(loaf)	(roll) ◯
Kaiser	(loaf)	(roll) ◯	**Rye**	(loaf) ◯	(roll)
Knot, double	(loaf)	(roll) ◯			

(Continued)

Activity C ***(Continued)*** **Name** ____________________________

Part 3: Proofing and Baking

Circle the clue in parentheses that best completes each of the following statements.

11. Proofing is complete when (**the dough doubles in size**) (**the end size of the product is reached**) (**two and a half hours have passed**).
12. When proofing is complete, the dough may be coated with a liquid to (**stop the gluten**) (**give the dough a particular color or create a textured crust**) (**to add to the taste of the product**).
13. Docking at the end of proofing creates a decorative pattern on a finished loaf and also allows (**the crust on soft crust breads to keep its shape**) (**gases to escape on hard crust breads during the baking process**).
14. At the (**beginning**) (**middle**) (**end**) of the baking process, the dough rises due to the expansion of the gases present in the dough.
15. During the baking process, yeast is (**activated**) (**stabilized**) (**killed**).
16. During the baking process, moisture in the dough (**evaporates**) (**condenses**) (**increases**).
17. During the baking process, starches and gluten in the dough (**evaporate**) (**become soft**) (**become firm**).

Pies and Tarts 44

Terminology

Chapter 44
Activity A

Name ____________________________
Date ____________ **Period** ____________

Match the following terms and identifying statements. Terms may be used more than once.

Answer	Statement
F	1. A very flaky dough made by a process that creates over 1,000 extremely thin layers of dough and fat.
E	2. A commercially prepared product made from fruit jelly and gelatin.
H	3. Also called *pâte sucrée.*
A	4. Prebaking a pie or tart shell.
C	5. Dough in which the fat is cut into the flour until it has the texture of cornmeal.
G	6. Also called *pâte brisée.*
B	7. Dough in which the fat is cut into the flour until it is in pieces approximately the size of a pea.
F	8. Has the richest taste and flakiest texture of all baked goods.
A	9. Pie and tart shells are typically weighted down during this process.
C	10. Is the best choice of dough for pies with liquid fillings.
G	11. A dough used for savory tarts.
H	12. Dough that contains sugar and egg yolks and may contain flavorings such as ground nuts.
D	13. The results from the way the ingredients are combined in a pie—neither extraordinary nor great.

A. blind baking
B. flaky pie dough
C. mealy pie dough
D. mediocre
E. pastry glaze
F. puff pastry
G. short dough
H. sweet dough

Preparing Quality Dough for Pies and Tarts

Chapter 44 **Name** ___________________________

Activity B **Date** __________ **Period** __________

Circle the clue in parentheses that best completes each of the following statements.

1. Most bakers use pastry flour for piecrusts because pastry flour is (**lower in gluten and higher in starch**) (**higher in gluten and lower in starch**) (**lower in gluten and lower in starch**) (**higher in gluten and higher in starch**).
2. The key to choosing the best fat for creating excellent texture is the (**weight**) (**melting point**) (**liquidity**) of the fat.
3. The best fat for creating flaky texture in the finished pie is (**liquid fat**) (**solid shortening**).
4. Crusts made with butter are (**more flaky than**) (**just as flaky as**) (**not as flaky as**) crusts made with shortening.
5. It is important that the liquid used in pie dough be (**hot**) (**lukewarm**) (**cool**) (**ice cold**).
6. To make flaky pie dough, the fat is mixed or cut into the flour until it (**resembles the texture of cornmeal**) (**is in pieces about the size of a pea**).
7. To make mealy pie dough, the fat is mixed or cut into the flour until it (**resembles the texture of cornmeal**) (**is in pieces about the size of a pea**).
8. All types of pie dough should not be overworked to avoid developing (**too much**) (**too little**) gluten.
9. When rolling out dough, make sure the temperature of the dough is (**hot**) (**warm**) (**cold**).
10. When you are making multiple pies, it (**is**) (**is not**) a good idea to roll out more than one crust at a time.
11. About (**six**) (**nine**) (**twelve**) ounces of dough is enough to line a standard nine-inch pie pan.
12. Dough is typically rolled out to about (**1/16-inch**) (**1/8-inch**) (**1/4-inch**) thickness.
13. Dough is dusted with flour during rolling to keep the dough (**dry**) (**from sticking**) (**from falling apart**).
14. As dough is rolled out it should (**not be turned**) (**periodically be turned 90 degrees**).

Reviewing Key Concepts

Chapter 44 **Name** ______________________________

Activity C **Date** ___________ **Period** ___________

Part 1: Fillings for Pies

Read each statement below. Circle the letter *T* if the statement is true. If the statement is false, circle *F* and write the corrected statement on the lines that follow.

T (F) 1. Most commercial operations prepare fruit filling for pies with raw fruit, which is the most traditional way of preparing fruit pies.

Most commercial operations prepare cooked fruit filling for pies.

(T) F 2. When using cooked fillings involving delicate fruit, just the juice is sweetened and thickened on the stove top.

T (F) 3. Most liquid fillings contain no ingredient that can thicken the filling.

Most liquid fillings contain eggs that coagulate and thicken the filling.

T (F) 4. Cream pies require baking.

Cream pies do not require baking.

(T) F 5. It is essential to use a prebaked pie shell or crumb crust pie shell for chiffon pies.

T (F) 6. Chiffon pies are essentially cream fillings to which whipped cream and butter have been added.

Chiffon pies are essentially cream fillings to which whipped cream and gelatin have been added.

(Continued)

Activity C *(Continued)* **Name** ______________________

T (F) 7. Some common examples of liquid fillings are custard, pumpkin, and Bavarian cream.

Some common examples of liquid fillings are custard, pumpkin, and pecan pies.

(T) F 8. Mealy crusts are best for liquid fillings.

____

____

Part 2: Tarts

Circle the clue in parentheses that best completes each of the following statements.

9. The nature of the pastry crust for tarts is essentially the same except that tarts are (**shallower**) (**deeper**) than pies.
10. The classical shape for tarts is (**round**) (**oval**) (**square**) (**rectangular**).
11. Traditionally, the sides of tarts are (**straight**) (**fluted**).
12. Short dough is a dough similar to (**flaky**) (**mealy**) pie dough.
13. Sweet dough is a dough similar to (**flaky**) (**mealy**) (**short**) dough.
14. Tart dough that contains egg yolks is (**short**) (**sweet**).
15. The dough used for savory tart fillings is (**short**) (**sweet**) dough.
16. The dough used for sweet tart fillings is (**short**) (**sweet**) dough.
17. The most common filling for sweet dough tarts is (**whipped cream**) (**pastry cream**).
18. Pastry glaze is brushed on fresh fruit tart toppings to (**make it shiny**) (**keep the fruit from drying out**).
19. The most common flavor of pastry glaze used in bakeshops is (**cherry**) (**apple**) (**apricot**) (**peach**) (**orange**).

(Continued)

Activity C *(Continued)* Name ______________________

Part 3: Puff Pastry

Answer the following questions about puff pastry in the space provided.

20. Once a basic dough made with flour, butter, and water is prepared, what steps are taken to turn the basic dough into puff pastry?

    A layer of butter is spread on the dough; the dough is folded and rolled out; the process of folding and rolling the dough is repeated multiple times to create many layers of fat in the dough.

21. Why do many foodservice operations buy ready-made puff pastry?

    Because making puff pastry is so labor intensive.

22. What kinds of fillings can be used with puff pastry?

    Both sweet and savory fillings can be used with puff pastry.

23. How does puff pastry relate to menu items described as *en croute*?

    A product baked in pastry crust (en croute) is usually baked in puff pastry.

24. How does puff pastry relate to the classic dessert *napoleon*?

    Puff pastry is layered with pastry cream to create the classic dessert called a *napoleon*.

Notes

Cakes 45

The Chemical Properties of Cake Ingredients

Chapter 45
Activity A

Name ______________________
Date ___________ Period ___________

Complete the chart by circling the function of each ingredient and indicating the specific properties that ingredient provides. Use the corresponding letters from the list that follows to complete the *Properties* column.

Cake Ingredients			
Ingredient	**Function** ***(circle one)***		**Properties** ***(from list)***
Egg	(gives structure)	tenderizes	C, G
Flour	(gives structure)	tenderizes	I, K
Liquid	(gives structure)	tenderizes	A, E, F
Shortening	gives structure	(tenderizes)	B, H
Sweetener	gives structure	(tenderizes)	D, J

A. Aids in gluten development when mixed with flour.

B. Adds richness to the cake, and, depending on specific product, may add flavor.

C. Acts as the main source of leavening for many cakes.

D. Helps absorb liquid, which contributes to a moist cake.

E. Helps create steam for leavening in the baking process.

F. Helps dissolve sugar.

G. Incorporates air and gives light, airy texture to product.

H. Prevents overdevelopment of gluten.

I. Its proteins coagulate trapping moisture and gases.

J. Provides a sweet taste.

K. Its starch absorbs moisture.

Classifying Cakes by Mixing Methods

Chapter 45 Name ______________________

Activity B Date __________ Period __________

Cakes are typically mixed using one of two methods—*creaming* or *sponge*. Write the mixing method that best matches each description. If the statement refers to both methods, write both terms.

Description	Mixing Method
1. creaming	Method used for cakes with a high proportion of butter or shortening.
2. sponge	Begins with combining the egg products with some or all of the sugar.
3. sponge	Method used for genoise.
4. creaming	Starts by mixing the butter or shortening with the sugar in an electric mixer with the paddle attachment
5. sponge	Leavened by air whipped into eggs in the cake formula.
6. creaming	After shortening is mixed with sugar, eggs and liquid are added.
7. creaming, sponge	The second step in this method is to preheat the oven and prepare cake pans.
8. creaming	Eggs are added gradually in this method.
9. sponge	This method is also called the *foam method*.
10. creaming	Dry ingredients are added last in this method.
11. sponge	In this method, eggs and sugar are whipped at high speed to incorporate air.
12. sponge	In this method, liquid or melted fat is added last.
13. creaming, sponge	Care must be taken to not overmix cake batter when using this method.
14. creaming, sponge	Batter prepared by this method, must be portioned into pans and baked immediately.
15. sponge	Eggs and sugar are beaten until they are thick and ribbonlike.
16. sponge	Method used for cakes with a high proportion of eggs to flour.

Reviewing Key Concepts

Chapter 45 Name ____________________

Activity C Date __________ Period __________

Part 1: Preparing a Cake Pan and Baking

Circle the clue in parentheses that best completes each of the following statements.

1. Pans can be brushed with (**solid**) (**liquid**) (**solid or liquid**) shortening and then dusted with (**flour**) (**sugar**) (**flour or sugar**). Excess dusting ingredient (**will be absorbed when**) (**should be shaken out before**) the batter is poured in.
2. An alternative to dusting is to line the pan with (**plastic wrap**) (**parchment paper**).
3. The most common method used to determine the doneness of a cake is to use a skewer or toothpick. When a skewer or toothpick is inserted into the center of a baked cake, it should come out (**with dry crumbs clinging to it**) (**with moist crumbs clinging to it**) (**clean**).
4. Bakers may test a cake for doneness by gently pressing the cake. The cake is done if (**it leaves a small indent**) (**the cake springs back**).
5. A visual sign of doneness is when the sides of the cake (**darken**) (**pull away from the sides of the pan**) (**puff over the sides of the pan**).

Part 2: Assembling and Finishing Layer Cakes

Read each statement below. Circle the letter *T* if the statement is true. If the statement is false, circle *F* and write the corrected statement on the lines that follow.

T F 6. Cakes should be flipped so the top of the cake is the smooth surface created from the bottom of the cake pan.

____

____

T F 7. To split cakes into layers, use a chef's knife.

To split cakes into layers, use a serrated knife.

____

(Continued)

Activity C *(Continued)* **Name** ______________________

(T) F 8. Before filling the layers, it is common to brush the layers with simple syrup to create a moist cake and add sweetness.

____

____

T (F) 9. To assemble layers, a thick coating of filling should be placed on the bottom layer of cake, and the next layer should be placed on top.

To assemble layers, a thin coating of filling should be placed on the bottom layer of cake, and the next layer should be placed on top.

T (F) 10. The most popular icings are buttercream and sour cream.

The most popular icings are buttercream and whipped cream.

____

T (F) 11. A pattern is often made on the sides of a cake by holding a pastry brush against the side of the cake at an angle and applying slight pressure while rotating the turntable.

A pattern is often made on the sides of a cake by holding a pastry comb against the side of the cake at an angle and applying slight pressure while rotating the turntable.

(T) F 12. Crumbs of nuts, shaved chocolate, or confections may be used to decorate sides of cakes.

____

____

(T) F 13. Icings in a pastry bag are used to create patterns on cakes and around the base of cakes.

____

____

Custards, Foams, and Buttercreams 46

Terminology

Chapter 46 **Name** ____________________

Activity A **Date** ______ **Period** __________

Match the following terms and identifying statements. Terms may be used more than once.

D 1. Pastry cream to which whipped cream has been added.

G 2. Stable foam dessert that is solidified by fat or gelatin and lightened with whipped cream and sometimes Italian meringue.

B 3. Custard sauce that, in addition to being used as a sauce, is the base of important preparations such as Bavarian cream and many ice creams.

F 4. Foam made by beating egg whites with sugar.

I 5. Name of the process that gently raises the temperature of the egg yolks to prevent curdling.

A 6. A stable foam dessert made from crème anglaise that is bound with gelatin and lightened with whipped cream.

H 7. Sweetened milk that is thickened with starch and egg yolks.

C 8. Classical name for sweetened whipped cream.

G 9. The French word that means *foam*.

H 10. Its French name, commonly used in many kitchens, is *crème pâtissière*.

B 11. Is thickened solely by egg yolks, and must not be boiled during preparation.

E 12. To introduce flavors into milk before the tempering process.

A. Bavarian cream
B. crème anglaise
C. crème chantilly
D. crème mousseline
E. infuse
F. meringue
G. mousse
H. pastry cream
I. tempering

Various Forms of Custards and Foams

Chapter 46 Name ______________________

Activity B Date __________ Period __________

Part 1: Custards

Circle the clue in parentheses that best completes each of the following statements.

1. Stirred custards are prepared (**in the oven**) (**on the stovetop**).
2. Pastry cream is prepared (**in the oven**) (**on the stovetop**).
3. Crème anglaise is prepared (**in the oven**) (**on the stovetop**).
4. Pastry cream is also known as (**custard**) (**mousse**) (**crème mousseline**).
5. Pastry cream is sweetened milk thickened with (**starch and egg yolks**) (**starch**) (**egg yolks**) (**beaten egg whites**).
6. Pastry cream is considered a potentially hazardous food because it (**can be a breeding ground for pathogens**) (**it has a high fat content**).
7. Pastry cream is generally flavored with (**almond**) (**cinnamon**) (**vanilla**), but other flavors can be used as well.
8. Adding whipped cream to pastry cream creates (**crème anglaise**) (**crème mousseline**) (**Bavarian cream**).
9. Pastry cream has the consistency of (**thick pudding**) (**thick sauce**) (**thin sauce**).
10. In addition to its use as a sauce, (**crème anglaise**) (**mousse**) (**crème mousseline**) is the base of preparations such as Bavarian cream and many ice creams.
11. Crème anglaise is thickened solely by (**egg yolks**) (**starch**) (**gelatin**).
12. (**Pastry cream**) (**Crème anglaise**) must always be boiled.
13. (**Pastry cream**) (**Crème anglaise**) must never be boiled.
14. When preparing crème anglaise professional chefs know that the product is done when it is thick enough to coat the (**tines of a metal fork**) (**back of a wooden spoon**) or reaches a temperature between 180°F and 185°F (82°C and 85°C).
15. If crème anglaise (**gets too hot**) (**does not get hot enough**) the yolks do not thicken properly and the finished product is thin and watery.
16. If crème anglaise (**gets too hot**) (**does not get hot enough**) it will separate.
17. To help moderate the cooking process, (**baked custards**) (**stirred custards**) (**all custards**) are placed in a bain marie in the oven.

(Continued)

Activity B *(Continued)* **Name** ______________________________

Part 2: Foams

Circle the clue in parentheses that best completes each of the following statements.

18. Whipped cream is lightened by (**egg whites**) (**gelatin**) (**air**).
19. Preferably, whipped cream is made from cream with a (**25%**) (**36%**) (**40%**) butterfat level.
20. One important rule when making whipped cream is to keep the cream (**cold**) (**warm**).
21. Most whipped cream is used between the (**very soft and soft**) (**soft and firm**) (**firm and stiff**) peak stages.
22. Adding sugar to whipped cream when the cream reaches the soft peak stage creates (**crème anglaise**) (**crème chantilly**) (**crème mousseline**).
23. Meringue is a foam made by beating (**egg whites**) (**egg yolks**) (**gelatin**) with sugar.
24. Overwhipping will destroy (**meringue**) (**whipped cream**) (**meringue and whipped cream**).
25. Properly made meringue is a(n) (**unstable**) (**stable**) foam.
26. Meringue made by combining all of the sugar and egg whites at once, cooking the mixture over boiling water, and then whipping it to firm peak stage is (**French meringue**) (**Swiss meringue**) (**Italian meringue**).
27. Meringue made by adding some of the sugar at the soft peak stage and then whipping the mixture to the firm peak stage, at which time the rest of the sugar is folded in is (**French meringue**) (**Swiss meringue**) (**Italian meringue**).
28. Meringue made by preparing a hot sugar and water syrup which is slowly poured into the egg whites as they are beaten at high speed is (**French meringue**) (**Swiss meringue**) (**Italian meringue**).
29. Two meringues that are generally piped into various shapes and baked at a low temperature are (**French and Swiss**) (**French and Italian**) (**Swiss and Italian**) meringue.
30. (**Mousse**) (**Bavarian cream**) (**Mousse and Bavarian cream**) is/are solidified by fat or gelatin and lightened with whipped cream and sometimes Italian meringue.
31. (**Mousse**) (**Bavarian cream**) (**Mousse and Bavarian cream**) is/are made from crème anglaise that is bound with gelatin and lightened with whipped cream.
32. (**Mousse**) (**Bavarian cream**) (**Mousse and Bavarian cream**) can be served alone or combined with other ingredients such as cake or fruit to make complex desserts.

Buttercreams

Chapter 46 **Name** ____________________

Activity C **Date** __________ **Period** __________

Characteristics of buttercreams are listed in the left column of the chart below. Place a check (✓) in column that corresponds with the type of buttercream—American or French—being described. Some characteristics may require a check in both columns.

Comparison of Buttercreams		
	American	**French**
Consists of egg yolks, sugar syrup, and butter.		✓
Consists of softened butter and a large amount of powdered sugar.	✓	
Is very sweet.	✓	
Is less sweet.		✓
Is less stable in hot environments.		✓
Is very stable even in hot conditions.	✓	
Is the preference of many pastry shops because it is the easiest to prepare.	✓	
Is somewhat complicated to make.		✓
Is often referred to as frosting.	✓	
Has a higher fat content.		✓
Can be flavored in many ways with the addition of extracts or melted chocolate.	✓	✓
Once it is homogenous, it is ready to be used.	✓	✓
If it is not used immediately, it should be refrigerated.	✓	✓

Dessert Sauces and Frozen Desserts

47

Culinary Terminology

Chapter 47 **Name** ____________________

Activity A **Date** __________ **Period** __________

Match the following terms and identifying statements. Terms may be used more than once.

Answer	Statement
B	1. Fruit sauces that are a mixture of puréed fruit, simple syrup, and, sometimes lemon juice.
D	2. A mixture made by combining chopped chocolate and boiling hot heavy cream.
A	3. This preparation should not be stirred as it cooks.
E	4. A slightly less-sweet style of sorbet.
H	5. A cross between sorbet and ice cream.
I	6. French name for a frozen mixture of fruit purée, sugar, and water.
C	7. Instrument that measures the sugar levels in fruit purées and syrups.
G	8. The name for the air that is frozen in ice cream.
A	9. Sugar that is cooked to about 320°F (160°C).
G	10. Adding high amounts of this to ice cream lowers the quality of the ice cream.
D	11. Once cooled, can be used for pastry specialties such as chocolate truffles and cake fillings and coverings.
B	12. The quality of this sauce is dependent on the quality of the fruit used.
H	13. A coulis-type mixture with the addition of a dairy product.
F	14. Something well-known such as ganache.

A. caramel
B. coulis
C. densimeter
D. ganache
E. granité
F. notable
G. overrun
H. sherbet
I. sorbet

Preparing Dessert Sauces and Frozen Desserts

Chapter 47 Name ____________________________

Activity B Date ___________ Period___________

Circle the clue in parentheses that best completes each of the following statements.

1. One method of making chocolate sauce is to bring water, milk, or cream to a boil; add chopped chocolate; and then (**turn down**) (**turn up**) (**remove from**) heat. Stir until the chocolate has (**melted**) (**solidified**) and the sauce is homogenous.

2. The other method of making chocolate sauce is to melt chocolate in a (**granité**) (**densimeter**) (**baine marie**), add heated (**liquid**) (**sugar**), and stir until the desired consistency is reached.

3. Crème anglaise is considered a classic dessert sauce because it is of (**pourable**) (**spreadable**) consistency.

4. Step one of making caramel sauce is (**boiling the water**) (**cooking the sugar**).

5. When making caramel sauce, the sugar should (**always**) (**occasionally**) (**never**) be stirred.

6. Step two of making caramel sauce is adding liquid to the caramel to (**cool it down**) (**thin it out**) (**dilute the flavor**).

7. The liquid most often added when making caramel sauce is (**cold water**) (**hot water**) (**cold cream**) (**hot cream**) but could also be (**cold water**) (**hot water**) (**cold cream**) (**hot cream**).

8. Fruit sauces are the (**most difficult**) (**easiest**) sauces to make.

9. Fruit sauces are most often a mixture of puréed fruit, (**coulis**) (**powdered sugar**) (**simple syrup**), and lemon juice if needed.

10. If peaches and pears are not cooked before blending, they will (**be too hard**) (**turn brown**) (**spoil**).

11. Frozen fruit purées (**should never**) (**may be**) used as a substitute for fresh fruit in fruit sauces.

12. If a fruit sauce is too thick, (**water**) (**appropriate juice**) (**either water or appropriate juice**) is generally added to adjust the consistency.

13. Traditional ice cream begins with (**coulis**) (**ganache**) (**crème anglaise**).

(Continued)

Activity B *(Continued)* **Name** ______________________

14. As the amount of butterfat in ice cream increases, the richness and quality of the ice cream (**increases**) (**decreases**).

15. Any ice cream product that is less than (**10**) (**20**) (**30**) percent butterfat must be labeled light, low fat, or reduced fat.

16. The purpose of continually churning ice cream as it freezes is to help (**form large ice crystals**) (**prevent the formation of large ice crystals**).

17. Air added to ice cream during mixing contributes to (**ice crystal formation**) (**a light texture**) (**a grainy texture**).

18. Ice creams that begin with crème anglaise are also called (**French**) (**eggless**) (**fruit**) ice creams.

19. Sorbet is most closely related to (**crème anglaise**) (**coulis**) (**ganache**).

20. The more sugar a sorbet contains, the (**softer**) (**harder**) the finished sorbet will be.

21. A granité is a style of sorbet that is often slightly (**more**) (**less**) sweet than regular sorbet.

22. Sherbet is a cross between (**ice cream and granité**) (**ice cream and sorbet**) (**granité and sorbet**).

Reviewing Key Concepts

Chapter 47 **Name** ____________________

Activity C **Date** __________ **Period** __________

Read each statement below. Circle the letter *T* if the statement is true. If the statement is false, circle *F* and write the corrected statement on the lines that follow.

(T) F 1. Dessert sauces contribute flavor and moisture, as well as improve the appearance of a dessert.

T (F) 2. When adding cream to hot caramel, the cream should be added all at once.

When adding cream to hot caramel, the cream should be added slowly a little at a time.

T (F) 3. Once crème anglaise is cooled, it can be used to make truffles.

Once ganache is cooled, it can be used to make truffles.

T (F) 4. Chocolate sauce shouldn't have flavors added because chocolate has a distinctive flavor.

Chocolate sauce can be flavored in a number of ways.

T (F) 5. If the caramel browns irregularly when making caramel sauce, gently stir the sugar.

If the caramel browns irregularly when making caramel sauce, swirl the pan over heat and never stir.

(T) F 6. If portions of a caramel sauce form lumps that do not dissolve, bring the mixture to a boil and stir until smooth.

T (F) 7. The quality of a coulis depends on the quantity of sugar.

The quality of a coulis depends on the quality of fruit used.

(Continued)

Activity C ***(Continued)*** **Name** ______________________

(T) F 8. *Overrun* is the name for air that is frozen in ice cream.

____

____

(T) F 9. Sorbet is a frozen mixture of fruit purée, sugar, and water.

____

____

T (F) 10. The amount of water in sorbet determines the texture of the finished sorbet.

The amount of sugar in sorbet determines the texture of the finished sorbet.

____

T (F) 11. The proportion of water, puréed fruit, and sugar in sorbet is standard for all types of fruit sorbet.

The proportion of water, puréed fruit, and sugar in sorbet varies depending on the type of fruit used.

(T) F 12. A granité is a coulis that is allowed to freeze in a shallow pan and is stirred from time to time as it freezes.

____

____

T (F) 13. Legally, sherbet must contain between 5 to 10 percent butterfat.

Legally, sherbet must contain between 1 to 2 percent butterfat.

____

T (F) 14. Densimeters measure the moisture levels in fruit purées and syrups using the brix or baumé scales.

Densimeters measure the sugar levels in fruit purées and syrups using the brix or baumé scales.

Notes

Table Service 48

Terminology

Chapter 48
Activity A

Name ______________________

Date __________ **Period** __________

Match the following terms and identifying statements.

A 1. Style of service in which the server delivers plates of food from the kitchen to the guest.

D 2. Style of service in which the waitperson places platters of prepared food in the center of the table and guests serve themselves.

K 3. A computer-based ordering system that transmits the order to the kitchen, produces the customer's bill, and keeps track of important data.

G 4. Style of service in which servers prepare dishes in front of the guests.

I 5. Dining room manager responsible for the entire dining room operations.

L 6. Style of service in which the front-of-house staff serves food from a platter onto preset plates in front of the guests.

B 7. Kitchen personnel.

J 8. Includes the china, flatware, glassware, and napkin used by one person.

F 9. The name for knives, forks, and spoons.

C 10. A tool used to scrape and scoop crumbs from the table.

H 11. Service personnel that work the dining room.

E 12. Refers to a dish that a server finishes by setting it aflame at tableside.

A. American service
B. back-of-the-house staff
C. crumber
D. family-style service
E. flambé
F. flatware
G. French service
H. front-of-the-house staff
I. maître d'hôtel
J. place setting
K. point-of-sale (POS) system
L. Russian service

The Front-of-the-House Staff

Chapter 48 **Name** ______________________________

Activity B **Date** ____________ **Period** ____________

Part 1: Positions

Match the positions with their descriptions of duties.

__B__ 1. Principally responsible for clearing dirty dishes, changing linens, and resetting tables. Is also responsible for butter, bread, and water service.

__C__ 2. Sometimes called *captain*. Welcomes guests, presents menus, takes orders, serves the food, provides beverage service, and is responsible for the bill. They must coordinate the needs of the guests with other front-of-the-house positions as well as the kitchen staff.

__F__ 3. Responsible for taking reservations and booking parties via the telephone and the Internet.

__A__ 4. Aids the front server and is responsible for coordinating timing with the chef and delivering food from the kitchen to the dining room.

__D__ 5. Welcomes the guests to the dining room and, in many restaurants, leads the guests to their table and manages the reservations.

__E__ 6. Is responsible for the entire dining room operation. This position is to the dining room what the chef is to the kitchen.

A. back server

B. busperson

C. front server

D. host

E. maître d'hôtel

F. reservationist

Part 2: Keys to Quality Service

For each key to quality service below, select the statement that is the best example of that skill and write the letter in the blank provided.

__C__ 7. **Hospitable**

A. Keeps visually checking the rest of the room for problems while trying to listen to what the customer is saying.

B. Maintains a reserved demeanor but is always coolly polite.

C. Maintains eye contact, is sincerely welcoming, and smiles a greeting.

(Continued)

Activity B ***(Continued)*** **Name** ______________________

__B__ 8. **Poised**

A. Helps the customers realize that they are not the only guests in the restaurant.

B. Has developed strategies for staying calm and confident even when problems arise.

C. Protects the front-of-the-house staff reputation by making sure that the guests are aware when problems are the fault of the back-of-the house staff.

__C__ 9. **Knowledgeable**

A. Is willing to take a guess at answering customers' questions, especially when the house is busy.

B. Honestly tells the guests that they just don't know the answer to a question, if that is the case.

C. Takes time to learn as much as possible about the food being served that day.

__A__ 10. **Sense of Timing**

A. Stays focused on what is happening in the dining room at all times, anticipates customer needs, and does a good job of prioritizing tasks.

B. Brings food promptly, whenever the kitchen has it ready.

C. Tries to coordinate two tables so that the job of serving both is easier.

(Continued)

Activity B *(Continued)* **Name** ______________________

B 11. **Communication Skills**

A. Anticipates customer questions and saves time by cutting in when he or she has the idea.

B. Uses nonverbal cues to let the customer know he or she is listening. Always allows the customer to finish what he or she has to say before responding.

C. Helps customers get to the point by showing that he or she is busy through body language and expression.

A 12. **Ability to "Read" the Customer**

A. Carefully considers verbal and nonverbal cues to determine how the customer wants to be treated by the server.

B. Treats all people alike regardless of their social status.

C. Honestly shows their own personality, whether it is formal or folksy, and consistently treats all guests according to that style. Takes time to help customers adjust to that style with humor when possible.

Reviewing Key Concepts

Chapter 48 **Name** ______________________

Activity C **Date** __________ **Period** __________

Part 1: Meal Service Styles

The four main styles of meal service are *American*, *family-style*, *French*, and *Russian*. Write the style of meal service that best matches each description.

Description	Style of Meal Service
1. An informal style of service common in restaurants and banquet halls across America.	family-style
2. Requires that the servers cook and prepare dishes in front of the customer.	French
3. The server delivers plates of food directly from the kitchen to the guest.	American
4. The server must learn to hold a large fork and spoon in their dominant hand and use them like a pair of tongs to serve food.	Russian
5. Food is served by front-of-the-house staff from a platter onto preset plates in front of guests.	Russian
6. Often called *tableside service*.	French
7. Is the norm in American restaurants and can be a formal or informal service style depending on the restaurant.	American
8. Waitperson places platters of prepared food on the table and guests serve themselves.	family-style

Part 2: Presetting the Dining Area

Circle the clue in parentheses that best completes each of the following statements.

9. When just prior to serving each course, the appropriate flatware and glassware are placed in front of each guest, the place setting is (**basic American**) (**à la carte**) (**banquet**).
10. A service that consists of a dinner plate, one or two forks, spoon, knife, water glass, any additional glassware, a butter knife, and bread and butter plate is (**basic American**) (**à la carte**) (**banquet**).
11. A setting that has all needed glassware and flatware on the table before people are seated is (**basic American**) (**à la carte**) (**banquet**).

(Continued)

Activity C *(Continued)* **Name** ____________________

Part 3: Serving Guests

Read each statement below. Circle the letter *T* if the statement is true. If the statement is false, circle *F* and write the corrected statement on the lines that follow.

T (F) 12. When pouring water in front of the guest, pour from the left of the customer.

When pouring water in front of the guest, pour from the right of the customer.

(T) F 13. Many restaurants fill water glasses only if requested by the guest.

____

____

(T) F 14. One clue that indicates the table is ready to order is when most guests have set their menus back on the table after looking at them.

____

____

T (F) 15. Plates of food are always transported from the kitchen to the dining room on a rolling cart pushed by the server.

Plates of food can be transported from the kitchen to the dining room on a rolling cart, carried by the server, or on a tray carried by the server.

T (F) 16. Once the food is served, the back servers are relieved of their responsibility.

Once the food is served, the front and back servers carefully monitor the progress of the table.

T (F) 17. About mid-meal, the front server should ask the customer if everything is to the customer's liking.

Shortly after the food is served, the front server commonly asks the customer if everything is to their liking.

T (F) 18. If the host is not known, the server should guess who the host is and present that person with the check.

If the host is not known, the server should place the check in the center of the table.

(Continued)

Activity C *(Continued)* **Name** ____________________

Part 4: Beverages

T (F) 19. Espresso is a combination of cappuccino and steamed milk.

Espresso is prepared by forcing hot water quickly and under pressure through finely ground coffee.

(T) F 20. Cappuccino is a combination of espresso, steamed milk, and milk foam.

____

____

T (F) 21. The finest teas are sold in bags.

The finest teas are sold loose leaf.

____

T (F) 22. If using tea bags, the customer is brought the tea and a small pot of warm water.

If using tea bags, the customer is brought the tea and a small pot of boiling hot water.

Notes

Managing Resources

49

Terminology

Chapter 49

Activity A

Name ____________________

Date ________ Period ________

Part 1

Match the following terms and identifying statements.

G 1. A specific amount of product to be kept on hand in order to maintain a sufficient supply from one delivery to the next.

I 2. A document listing the items, quantities ordered, and the agreed prices.

B 3. Refers to the amount of food product that remains after cleaning, cooking, or other preparation.

D 4. A list of the quantities of products and their prices that are being delivered.

F 5. What results when a business' expenses are greater than its sales.

J 6. The dollars received by a foodservice operation in payment for a meal.

A 7. Indicates the raw, unprepared product in the same form it is delivered from the vendor.

C 8. The cost of food used to make a menu item for a customer.

H 9. A business report that lists the sales and expenses incurred to make those sales during a given period of time.

E 10. A process for drawing products from food storage.

A. as purchased (AP)

B. edible portion (EP)

C. food cost

D. invoice

E. issuing

F. loss

G. par stock

H. profit and loss statement (P&L)

I. purchase order (PO)

J. sales

(Continued)

Activity A *(Continued)* **Name** ____________________

Part 2

D 11. Includes all the expenses involved in maintaining a foodservice staff.

H 12. The process of determining and recording the usable amount, or edible portion, of a product.

E 13. What results when a business' sales are greater than its expenses.

A 14. The costs incurred to prepare and serve the meal.

C 15. Predicting how many diners will be served during the coming meal period and what menu items they will order.

G 16. The ratio of EP to AP.

B 17. The portion of food sales that was spent on food expenses.

F 18. A formal written or electronic request from a foodservice department to the storeroom.

A. expenses
B. food cost percentage
C. forecast
D. labor cost
E. profit
F. requisition
G. yield percentage
H. yield test

Managing Costs

Chapter 49 **Name** ______________________

Activity B **Date** __________ **Period** __________

Part 1: Food Costs

Read each statement below. Circle the letter *T* if the statement is true. If the statement is false, circle *F* and write the corrected statement on the lines that follow.

(T) F 1. The goal of purchasing is to assure that the kitchen gets the right product at the right price in the right quantity.

T (F) 2. An inventory is taken by estimating the amounts of various food products in house.

An inventory is taken by physically counting the amounts of various food products in house.

T (F) 3. The prices of food products are generally stable and seldom change.

The prices of food products change regularly.

T (F) 4. Procedures for receiving food products are a matter of inspection and paying.

Procedures for receiving food products are a matter of inspection and verification.

(T) F 5. Procedures for receiving food also require checking foods for proper temperature.

T (F) 6. Shelf space is the key to product shelf life.

Temperature is the key to product shelf life.

T (F) 7. Product rotation ensures that the most recently purchased items are used first.

Product rotation ensures that the oldest purchased items are used first.

(Continued)

Activity B *(Continued)* **Name** ________________

T (F) 8. Theft of food products is most often committed by a restaurant's customers.

Theft of food products is most often committed by restaurant staff.

(T) F 9. Larger foodservice operations have a process for drawing products from food storage called *issuing*.

(T) F 10. Before cooks can begin their mise en place, the chef must forecast how many diners will be served during the coming meal period and what will be ordered.

(T) F 11. Chefs base their forecasts on past business statistics.

T (F) 12. The chef uses a profit and loss sheet to communicate the number of each menu item the staff should prepare for meal service.

The chef uses a production sheet to communicate the number of each menu item the staff should prepare for meal service.

(T) F 13. One reason to cost out a recipe is to aid in accurate menu pricing.

T (F) 14. Yield tests are done most frequently on the least expensive ingredients in the kitchen.

Yield tests are done most frequently on the most expensive ingredients in the kitchen.

T (F) 15. A yield test is the ratio of EP to AP.

A yield percentage is the ratio of EP to AP.

(Continued)

Activity B ***(Continued)*** **Name** ______________________________

Part 2: Labor Costs

Circle the clue in parentheses that best completes each of the following statements.

16. The most important tool in controlling (**overall**) (**labor**) (**food waste**) costs is the staff schedule.

17. Most operations schedule kitchen staff on a (**daily**) (**weekly**) (**monthly**) basis.

18. Before creating the schedule, the chef needs to forecast the expected (**volume of business**) (**cost of sales**) for the week.

19. The largest cost in most foodservice operations is (**food**) (**labor**).

20. The actual labor cost is kept in check best by (**enforcing**) (**overlooking**) rules regarding the time clock or time sheets.

21. If the amount of business forecasted doesn't materialize, chefs (**must accept the loss**) (**may adjust the staff schedule**).

22. All decisions in scheduling and pay rates must be in accordance with (**federal**) (**state**) (**federal and state**) laws.

Calculating Food and Labor Cost Percentage

Chapter 49 **Name** ______________________________

Activity C **Date** ____________ **Period** ____________

Part 1

Food cost percentage shows the portion of food sales that was spent on food expenses. It is an important measure of how well a chef is managing the kitchen operation. Use the following formula to solve the problems below. Show your work in the space provided.

Food costs ÷ Food sales = Food cost percentage

Example: During the month of May, ABC restaurant spent \$43,600 on food to prepare menu items, which generated \$119,900 in food sales. Use the formula to calculate ABC restaurant's food cost percentage.

Food costs ÷ Food sales = [quotient as a decimal] x 100 = Food cost percentage

\$43,600 ÷ \$119,900 = 0.3636 x 100 = 36.36% (round up to 36.4%)

1. A restaurant had food costs of \$28,300 and food sales of \$61,000 during January. What was their food cost percentage? ___46.4___%

2. A restaurant had food costs of \$34,400 and food sales of \$72,500 during March. What was their food cost percentage for March? ___47.4___%

3. In April, the restaurant in Problem 2 experienced a change. Food costs stayed the same, but food sales increased to \$81,200. What was their food cost percentage for April? ___42.4___%

(Continued)

Activity C *(Continued)* **Name** ______________________

4. Suppose that food costs for the restaurant in Problem 2 stayed the same in April, but sales decreased to $69,500. What would their food cost percentage be for April? ___49.5___%

5. Suppose instead that food costs for the restaurant in Problem 2 decreased in April to $32, 900 and sales stayed the same as in March. What would their food cost percentage be for April? ___45.4___%

6. If the restaurant in Problem 2 experienced an increase in food costs to $36,700 in April and food sales stayed the same as in March, what would their food cost percentage be for April? ___50.6___%

Part 2

Labor cost percentage measures the amount of food sales that an establishment spent on labor during a specific period of time. Remember, labor costs include the cost of payroll, payroll taxes, and employee benefits. Use the following formula to solve the problems below. Show your work in the space provided.

Labor costs ÷ Food sales = Labor cost percentage

Example: During the month of May, ABC restaurant spent $37,500 on labor to prepare menu items that generated $119,900 in food sales. Use the formula to calculate ABC restaurant's labor cost percentage.

Labor costs ÷ Food sales = [quotient as a decimal] × 100 =Labor cost percentage

$37,500 ÷ $119,900 = 0.312 × 100 = 31.2%

7. A restaurant had labor costs of $27,700 and food sales of $75,000 during September. What is the restaurant's labor cost percentage? ___36.9___%

Activity C ***(Continued)*** **Name** ____________________

8. A restaurant had labor costs of $38,900 and food sales of $94,600 during October. What is the restaurant's labor cost percentage? 41.1 %

9. A restaurant had labor costs of $39,700 and food sales of $110,600 during November. What is the restaurant's labor cost percentage? 35.8 %

10. Suppose the restaurant in Problem 8 reduced labor costs to $36,600 in November but the food sales remained the same as October. What is the restaurant's labor cost percentage? 38.6 %

11. In December, the restaurant in Problem 9 experienced a change. Labor costs remained the same, but food sales increased to $117,700. What is the restaurant's labor cost percentage for December? 33.7 %

12. A restaurant is projecting January sales of $93,650. If the goal is to maintain labor cost percentage at 34%, how many dollars can be allocated for labor in January? $31,841

Part 3

Circle the clue in parentheses that best completes each of the following statements.

13. If food costs stay constant and sales increase, food cost percentage **(increases)** **(stays the same)** **(decreases)**.

14. If food costs stay constant and sales decrease, food cost percentage **(increases)** **(stays the same)** **(decreases)**.

15. If food costs decrease and sales stay constant, food cost percentage **(increases)** **(stays the same)** **(decreases)**.

16. If food costs increase and sales stay constant, food cost percentage **(increases)** **(stays the same)** **(decreases)**.

Nutrition 50

Terminology

Chapter 50 **Name** ____________________

Activity A **Date** __________ **Period** __________

Part 1

Match the following terms and identifying statements.

Answer	Statement	Term
F	1. Foods that have high nutritional value compared with the amount of calories they supply.	A. calorie
B	2. Chief energy source for the body.	B. carbohydrate
E	3. Are missing one or more of the nine indispensable amino acids.	C. complete protein
H	4. The way our body takes in and utilizes foods.	D. essential nutrients
A	5. Unit used to measure the amount of energy contained in foods.	E. incomplete protein
D	6. Nutrients that the body cannot make, and therefore must be supplied by diet.	F. nutrient-dense food
G	7. Substances in food that nourish the body.	G. nutrients
I	8. Substances produced by plants that may provide health benefits for humans.	H. nutrition
C	9. Contain all nine indispensable amino acids in the correct proportions needed to support life.	I. phytochemicals
L	10. Type of lipid that is created when unsaturated oil is chemically changed to resemble a saturated fat.	J. prebiotics
K	11. Foods containing live, beneficial bacteria that help counteract the "bad" bacteria in the gut.	K. probiotics
J	12. Nondigestible food products that encourage the growth of good bacteria in the gut.	L. *trans* fat

(Continued)

Activity A *(Continued)* **Name** ______________________

Part 2

__G__ 13. A type of fat that is solid at room temperature.

__B__ 14. White, pasty substance found in the bloodstream and cells that is essential for many body functions.

__D__ 15. The scientific term for fats.

__F__ 16. A molecule made up of a chain of various amino acids linked together in a particular order.

__C__ 17. Chemical process that changes liquid oil into solid fat.

__H__ 18. A type of fat that is liquid at room temperature.

__E__ 19. To prevent.

__A__ 20. Forces that hold chains of carbon atoms together.

A. bonds
B. cholesterol
C. hydrogenation
D. lipids
E. preclude
F. protein
G. saturated fat
H. unsaturated fat

The Role of Nutrients in Good Health

Chapter 50 Name ______________________________

Activity B Date ____________ Period____________

Circle the clue in parentheses that best completes each of the following statements.

1. The most energy-dense nutrient that humans consume is (**vitamins**) (**minerals**) (**protein**) (**lipids**) (**water**) (**carbohydrates**).
2. The nutrient that accounts for 50 to 60 percent of the weight of the human body is (**vitamins**) (**minerals**) (**protein**) (**lipids**) (**water**) (**carbohydrates**).
3. The nutrient that is referred to as the building blocks of the human body is (**vitamins**) (**minerals**) (**protein**) (**lipids**) (**water**) (**carbohydrates**).
4. The nutrient that ensures proper vision, supports the immune system, aids in the formation of healthy bones and teeth, and is part of the blood clotting process is (**vitamins**) (**minerals**) (**protein**) (**lipids**) (**water**) (**carbohydrates**).
5. The nutrient that is the body's chief energy source is (**vitamins**) (**minerals**) (**protein**) (**lipids**) (**water**) (**carbohydrates**).
6. The nutrient that is necessary for energy metabolism, bone formation, and proper functioning of the nervous system is (**vitamins**) (**minerals**) (**protein**) (**lipids**) (**water**) (**carbohydrates**).
7. The nutrient that is further classified as either fat soluble or water soluble is (**vitamins**) (**minerals**) (**protein**) (**lipids**) (**water**) (**carbohydrates**).
8. The nutrient that is part of skin, blood vessels, blood, inner organs, hair, nails, and enzymes is (**vitamins**) (**minerals**) (**protein**) (**lipids**) (**water**) (**carbohydrates**).
9. Saturated and unsaturated fats are part of the (**vitamins**) (**minerals**) (**protein**) (**lipids**) (**water**) (**carbohydrates**) nutrient group.
10. The nutrient that provides no energy but is part of almost all bodily functions is (**vitamins**) (**minerals**) (**protein**) (**lipids**) (**water**) (**carbohydrates**).
11. The nutrient that is further divided into major or trace categories is (**vitamins**) (**minerals**) (**protein**) (**lipids**) (**water**) (**carbohydrates**).
12. Fiber, which helps protect against some cancers and heart disease, is part of the (**vitamins**) (**minerals**) (**protein**) (**lipids**) (**water**) (**carbohydrates**) group of nutrients.

Dietary Guidelines

Chapter 50 Name ____________________

Activity C Date __________ Period__________

Answer the following.

1. Summarize the two overarching principles around which the *Dietary Guidelines for Americans* provide advice.

   Maintain calorie balance over time to achieve and sustain a healthy weight. Focus on consuming nutrient-dense foods and beverages.

2. What are nutrient-dense foods?

   Foods that provide vitamins, minerals, and other substances that may have beneficial health effects, but supply relatively few calories.

3. MyPlate divides commonly eaten foods into what five food groups?

   fruits, grains, vegetables, dairy, protein foods

4. Why should most of your fruit choices be whole or cut-up fruit rather than juice?

   Whole fruits supply fiber and are more nutrient dense than juice.

5. What amount of grains eaten should be whole grain?

   Half.

6. Into what subgroups is the vegetables group further divided? Give an example of each.

   (Answers include the following. Examples will vary.) dark green vegetables, red and orange vegetables, beans and peas, starchy vegetables, other vegetables

7. What nutrients do the foods in the dairy group provide?

   calcium, protein, potassium, and vitamin D

(Continued)

Activity C ***(Continued)*** **Name** ____________________

8. What recommendations does MyPlate make about choosing protein foods?

   Choose lean meats and poultry to limit saturated fats and cholesterol. Consume fish or seafood at least twice a week and incorporate plant-based proteins often.

9. What factors influence the amount of food a person should eat to meet energy needs?

   age, gender, weight, physical activity levels, health conditions, pregnancy

10. If energy needs increase, how do food amounts change? What other information do the Dietary Guidelines suggest?

    If energy needs increase, food amounts should also increase. The Guidelines suggest striving to select nutrient-dense foods more often.

Labeling and the Chef's Role

Chapter 50 Name ____________________

Activity D Date __________ Period__________

Part 1

Circle either ***required*** or ***voluntary*** to indicate whether each of the following items is required for ingredient labeling of foods.

required ***voluntary*** 1. A list of all ingredients in the product.

required ***voluntary*** 2. Ingredients listed in descending order by weight.

required ***voluntary*** 3. Content of each ingredient as a percentage of the whole.

required ***voluntary*** 4. Flavorings listed by their common names.

required ***voluntary*** 5. The name of the food source of any major food allergens contained in the product.

Part 2

Circle the clue in parentheses that best completes each of the following statements.

6. The first item on a nutrition label is (**amount of fat**) (**number of calories**) (**serving size**).
7. All the nutritional information listed on the Nutrition Facts panel is based on (**one serving**) (**two servings**) (**servings for a family of four**).
8. To the right of each nutrient listed on a Nutrition Facts panel is the percent Daily Values for all the nutrients except *trans* fat, sugar, and (**cholesterol**) (**sodium**) (**protein**).
9. The percent Daily Value is based on a (**1200-**) (**2000-**) (**2500-**) calorie diet.
10. The chef's role in promoting healthy eating is (**increasing**) (**staying the same**) (**decreasing**).
11. One way chefs influence the nutrition of diners is by choosing nutrient-dense foods, which are foods that (**are heavy by weight**) (**contain a variety of nutrients**) (**have high nutritional value for each calorie**).
12. Substituting healthy oils for saturated fats, steaming vegetables instead of boiling them, and trimming visible fats from meats are examples of the way that chefs influence the nutrition of diners by (**using healthy cooking techniques**) (**cutting calories**).
13. Restaurants typically (**do**) (**do not**) serve healthy ratios of protein to grains and vegetables.
14. Portion sizes in restaurants are typically (**too large**) (**too small**) (**just right**) because chefs are caught between the nutritional goal of (**smaller**) (**larger**) portions and the customers desire for value.

Accommodations for Special Needs

Chapter 50 Name ______________________

Activity E Date __________ Period __________

Part 1

Read each statement below about food allergies. Circle the letter *T* if the statement is true. If the statement is false, circle *F* and write the corrected statement on the lines that follow.

T (F) 1. A food allergy is a digestive system response.

A food allergy is an immune system response to a specific food.

(T) F 2. Symptoms of food intolerance may include nausea, vomiting, heartburn, headaches, or diarrhea.

(T) F 3. To help a customer identify dishes that may cause an allergic reaction, the waitstaff should understand how dishes are prepared and their ingredients.

T (F) 4. Because allergens are killed by cooking temperatures, the kitchen staff need not worry about transferring allergens from one dish to another.

Because allergens can often survive cooking temperatures, the kitchen staff must ensure that allergens are not transferred from one dish to another.

(T) F 5. To avoid transferring food allergens to food that does not normally contain these allergens, food handlers should wash hands and change gloves.

Activity E *(Continued)* **Name** ______________________

Part 2

Match the following terms and identifying phrases.

__E__ 6. People who eat no food from animal sources and limit their diets to plant-based foods only.

__B__ 7. People who eat milk, cheese, and other dairy products, but do not eat meat, fish, poultry, or eggs.

__C__ 8. People who do not eat meat, poultry, or dairy products, but who will eat eggs.

__A__ 9. People who eat dairy products and eggs, but do not consume meat, fish, or poultry.

__D__ 10. People who consume vegetables, fruits, nuts, beans, and fish or seafood, but exclude animal or poultry products.

A. Lacto-ovo vegetarian
B. Lacto vegetarian
C. Ovo vegetarian
D. Pescetarian
E. Vegan

Part 3

Answer the following.

11. How can individuals with health conditions meet their special needs with menu selections?

Individuals can choose fruits, vegetables, whole grains, lean meats and poultry, plant-based proteins, and fish and seafood from menu offerings. The can also make healthful selections with little or no added solid fat, salt, and sugar and served in moderate portion sizes.

12. What options might a person with heart disease or one who generally wants to manage his or her weight choose from a menu?

(Answers will vary, but may include:) broiled or grilled meats served without rich sauces, steamed or sautéed vegetables seasoned with lemon juice or vinegar, poached fish seasoned with herbs, seasonal fresh fruits for dessert, salads served with vinegar and oil dressing

51

Menus

Terminology

Chapter 51

Activity A

Name ______________________

Date __________ **Period** __________

Match the following terms and descriptive statements. Terms may be used more than once.

Answer	Statement
B	1. Menu format that rotates a set number of items over a certain period of time. After that time period, the daily menu offerings repeat.
D	2. Menu format that has one set price for the total meal but allows customers to make their own selection from each course offered.
F	3. Menu format that offers one set meal to all guests with no choices or substitutions.
C	4. Menu format composed daily based on what food products are available in the market that day.
A	5. Menu format that prices each course separately.
E	6. Menu format that offers the same items every day.
F	7. Today, a banquet is the most common use of this menu format.
A	8. A modified form of this menu format used in the United States prices each main course separately, but that price includes other courses such as soup or salad and accompaniments.
C	9. This menu format is most often found in fine-dining establishments.
C	10. This menu format allows chefs to use the best products available at any given time.
B	11. This menu format is effective in operations that serve the same customers day after day, such as schools and hospitals.
E	12. One disadvantage of this menu format is that repeat customers might become bored with the unchanging menu offerings.

A. à la carte menu
B. cycle menu
C. market menu
D. prix fixe menu
E. static menu
F. table d'hôte menu

Menu Planning

Chapter 51 **Name** ____________________

Activity B **Date** __________ **Period** __________

Read each statement below. Circle the letter *T* if the statement is true. If the statement is false, circle *F* and write the corrected statement on the lines that follow.

T (F) 1. The goal of good menu planning is to create a mix of menu items that satisfies diners at the lowest possible price.

The goal of good menu planning is to create a mix of menu items that satisfies diners while maximizing profits.

T (F) 2. The term *menu mix* refers to mixing the menu formats in a restaurant.

The term *menu mix* refers to the combination of items offered on a menu.

(T) F 3. In addition to pleasing the customers, it is important to choose a combination of menu items that distributes the workload in the kitchen.

T (F) 4. The ultimate goal of menu mix is a combination of items that generate the most sales at the lowest prices.

The ultimate goal of menu mix is a combination of items that generate the most sales at the greatest profits.

(T) F 5. The "going rate" is the price that competitors are charging for menu items.

T (F) 6. Competent operators base their menu price on the going rate of menu items.

Competent operators base their menu price on the actual cost of menu items.

(Continued)

Activity B *(Continued)* **Name** ______________________

T (F) 7. The simplest cost-based pricing method is the food cost percentage method.

The simplest cost-based pricing method is the markup method.

(T) F 8. The markup method involves adding a set amount to the cost of the menu item.

T (F) 9. The markup method is the most common method of setting menu prices.

Food cost percentage is the most common method of setting menu prices.

(T) F 10. The standard food cost percentage is determined during an operations financial planning and budgeting process.

Basing Price on Standard Food Cost Percentage

Chapter 51 **Name** ______________________

Activity C **Date** __________ **Period** __________

Foodservice operations commonly use the standard food cost percentage method to set menu prices. Use the following formula to complete the chart and answer the questions that follow. (Round answers up to nearest 25 cents, for example $6.02 rounds up to $6.25; $6.42 rounds up to $6.50; $6.80 rounds up to $7.00.)

Food cost per portion ÷ Standard food cost percentage = Menu price

Example: The manager of an operation that has established a 30% standard food cost needs to set a menu price for an appetizer portion of spring rolls. The recipe cost sheet performed on an appetizer portion of spring rolls shows a food cost per portion of $1.96.

Step 1. First convert the standard food cost percent to a decimal by moving the decimal point two places to the left.

30% = .30.0 = 0.30

Step 2. Calculate the menu price using the formula.

Food cost per portion ÷ Standard food cost percentage = Menu price

$1.96 ÷ 0.30 = $6.53 = (round up) $6.75

Food Item	Food Cost per Portion	Standard Food Cost Percentage	Menu Price
Green salad	$1.23	35%	$3.75
Lentil soup	$0.80	30%	$2.75
Beef entrée	$4.05	36%	$11.25
Fruit compote dessert	$1.67	32%	$5.25

1. If the restaurant above increased their standard food cost percentage to 32%, what would the new menu price for the lentil soup be?

   $2.50
2. If the same restaurant lowered their standard food cost percentage to 28%, what would the new menu price for the lentil soup be?

   $3.00
3. If a restaurant raises their standard food cost percentage, the menu price will (**increase**) (**decrease**) (**stay the same**).
4. If a restaurant lowers their standard food cost percentage, the menu price will (**increase**) (**decrease**) (**stay the same**).

Menu Mechanics

Chapter 51

Activity D

Name ______________________________

Date __________Period__________

Part 1

Circle the clue in parentheses that best completes each of the following statements.

1. Menu text should be accurate and (**colorful**) (**truthful**).
2. Menu text should be descriptive and as (**detailed**) (**brief**) as possible.
3. Menu text should avoid (**home-cooking terms**) (**culinary jargon**).
4. Menu text should be written in language (**that will most impress customers**) (**that customers can understand**).
5. Menu text should include the portion size of the main (**protein**) (**starch**) (**carbohydrate**) source.
6. Menu text should describe the (**finished look of the product**) (**cooking method**).
7. Menu text should highlight (**difficult processes**) (**unique ingredients**) that make the dish special.

Part 2

Complete the following list of elements to consider when planning menu design and layout.

8. Size, shape, and color of the menu card.
9. (answers can appear in any order:) type of paper
10. whether to use a holder or menu cover
11. layout or arrangement of items on the menu card
12. size, color, and typeface of menu text
13. illustrations and graphics to be used

Notes

Analyzing Cuisines

52

Terminology

Chapter 52 Name ______________________

Activity A Date ____________ Period ____________

Match the following terms and identifying phrases. Terms may be used more than once.

A 1. Something that is genuine.

F 2. A special set of characteristics in a food product that result from the local environment.

B 3. The eating habits and culinary practices of a people, region, or historical period.

D 4. Foods acceptable under Jewish dietary law.

E 5. To forbid something.

C 6. Foods acceptable in Islam.

D 7. A dietary custom in which no pork and only forequarter meats are consumed.

B 8. Historic events, trade routes, conquests, and occupations are factors that influence eating habits and culinary practices of a people.

F 9. Unique characteristics of ingredients from a specific place.

C 10. A dietary custom that requires meats be slaughtered according to ritual and forbids pork and alcohol.

D 11. A type of cooking that forbids mixing of meats and dairy foods.

A. authentic
B. foodways
C. halal
D. kosher
E. prohibit
F. terroir

Reviewing Key Concepts

Chapter 52 **Name** ______________________

Activity B **Date** __________ **Period** __________

Read each statement below. Circle the letter *T* if the statement is true. If the statement is false, circle *F* and write the corrected statement on the lines provided.

T (F) 1. Although there is greater demand for authentic cuisine, chefs require little knowledge and understanding of cuisines as long as they have quality recipes.

Because there is greater demand for authentic cuisine, chefs need to develop better knowledge and understanding of cuisines.

(T) F 2. Climate and geography are factors that influence terroir.

(T) F 3. Over time, when different ethnic groups living in the same region adopt and blend elements of each other's cuisines, *fusion cuisine* forms.

T (F) 4. One of the *least* important factors to understanding cuisine of a region or nation is understanding the basic food guidelines of major religious groups.

One of the *most* important factors in understanding cuisine to a region or nation is understanding the basic food guidelines of major religious groups.

T (F) 5. Religious practices seldom dictate what foods followers can and cannot eat, when they can eat them, or how they should prepare them.

Religious practices often dictate what foods followers can and cannot eat, when they can eat them, or how they should prepare them.

(T) F 6. To analyze a cuisine, chefs must break it down into its basic elements—ingredients, cooking methods, and dishes.

Identifying International and Regional Cuisines

Chapter 52 Name ______________________

Activity C Date __________ Period __________

For each of the regions listed in this activity, name four dishes. Then draw an arrow from the names of the dishes to the location on the maps where they are popular.

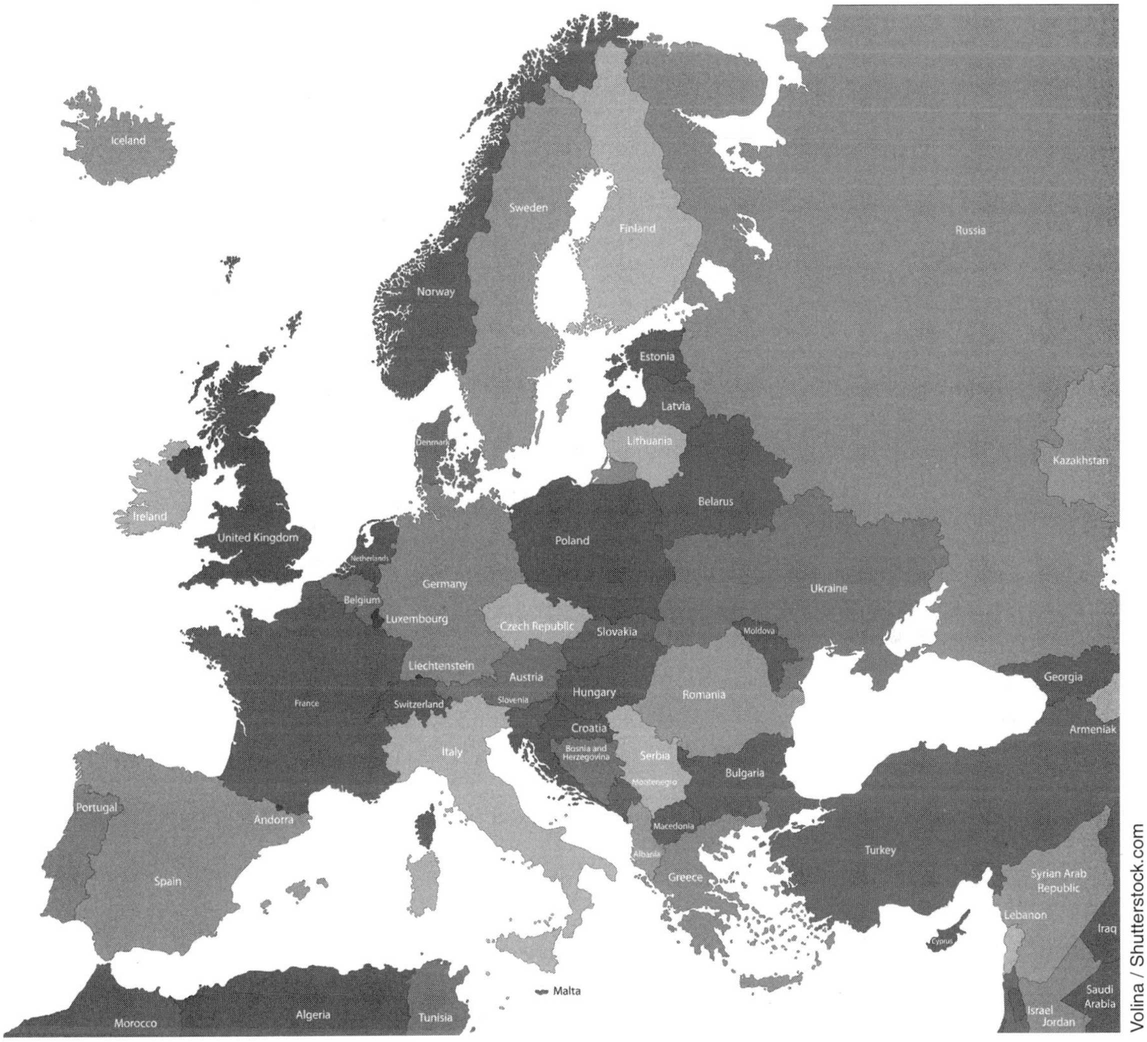

Western Europe

____

____

____

____

Central and Eastern Europe

____

____

____

____

(Continued)

Activity C *(Continued)* **Name** ______________________

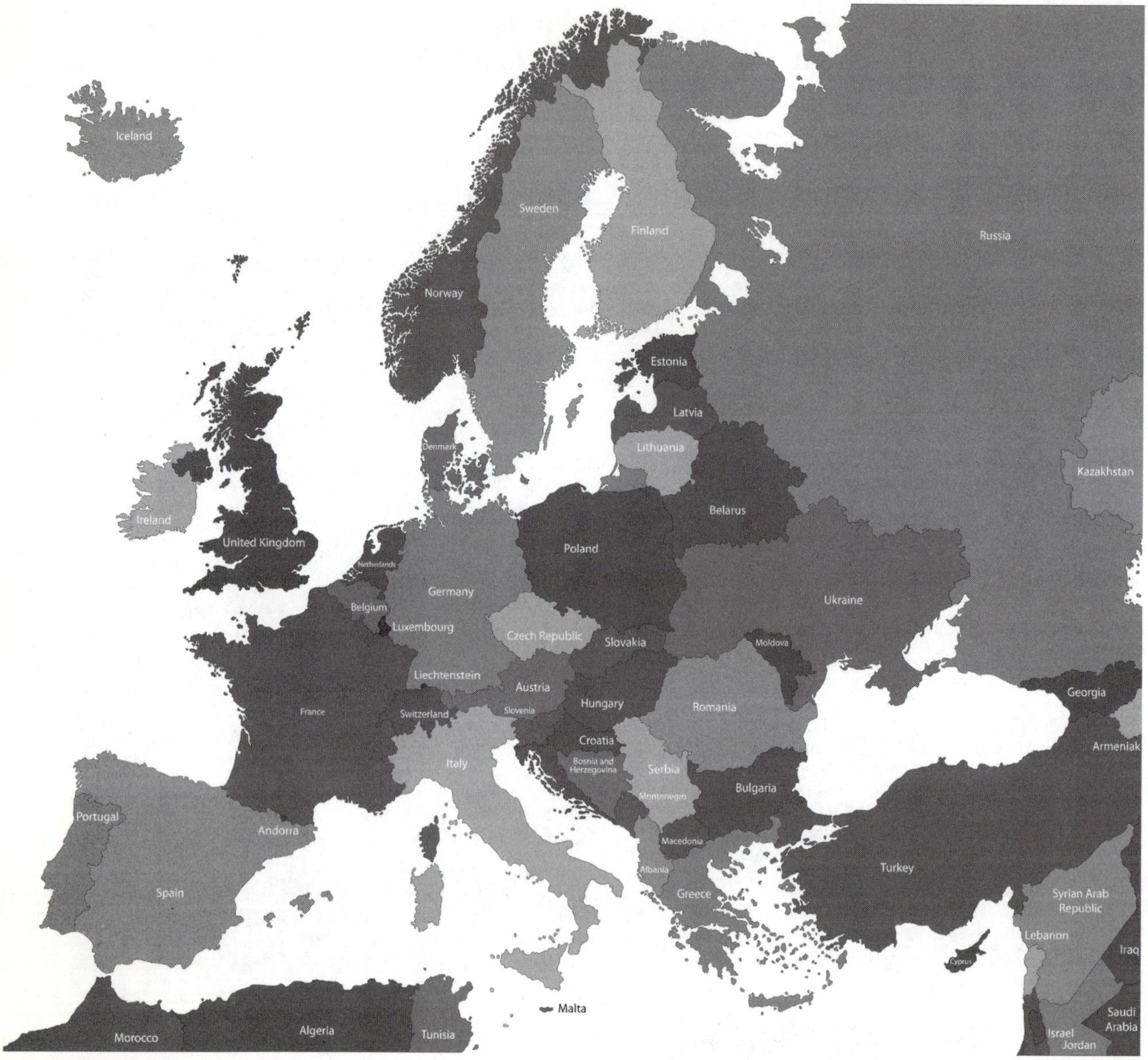

Volina / Shutterstock.com

Scandinavia

____

____

____

____

Mediterranean

____

____

____

____

(Continued)

Activity C *(Continued)* **Name** ______________________________

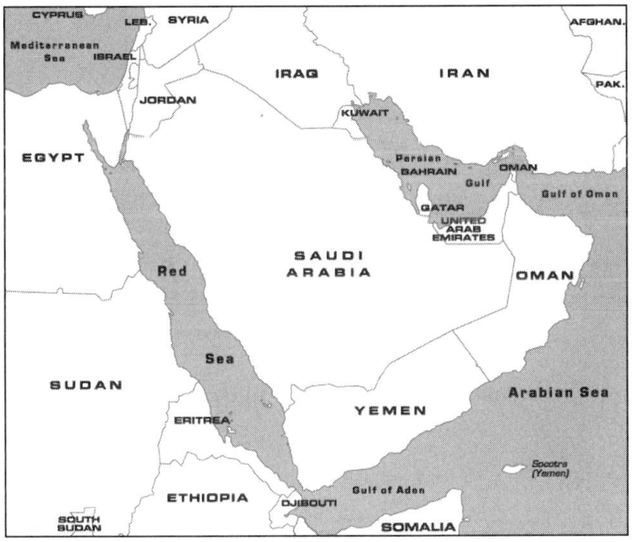

Globe Turner / Shutterstock.com

Middle East and Central Asia

____

____

____

____

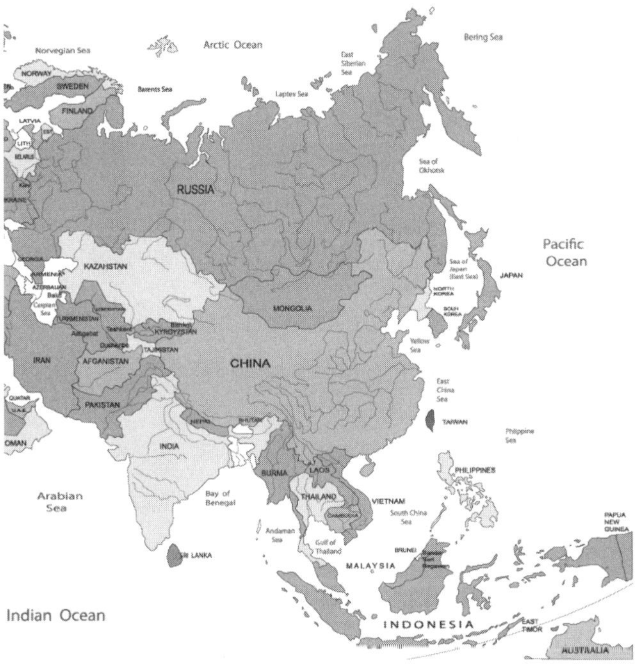

charobnica / Shutterstock.com

South Asia

____

____

____

____

East Asia

____

____

____

____

(Continued)

Activity C ***(Continued)*** **Name** ______________________

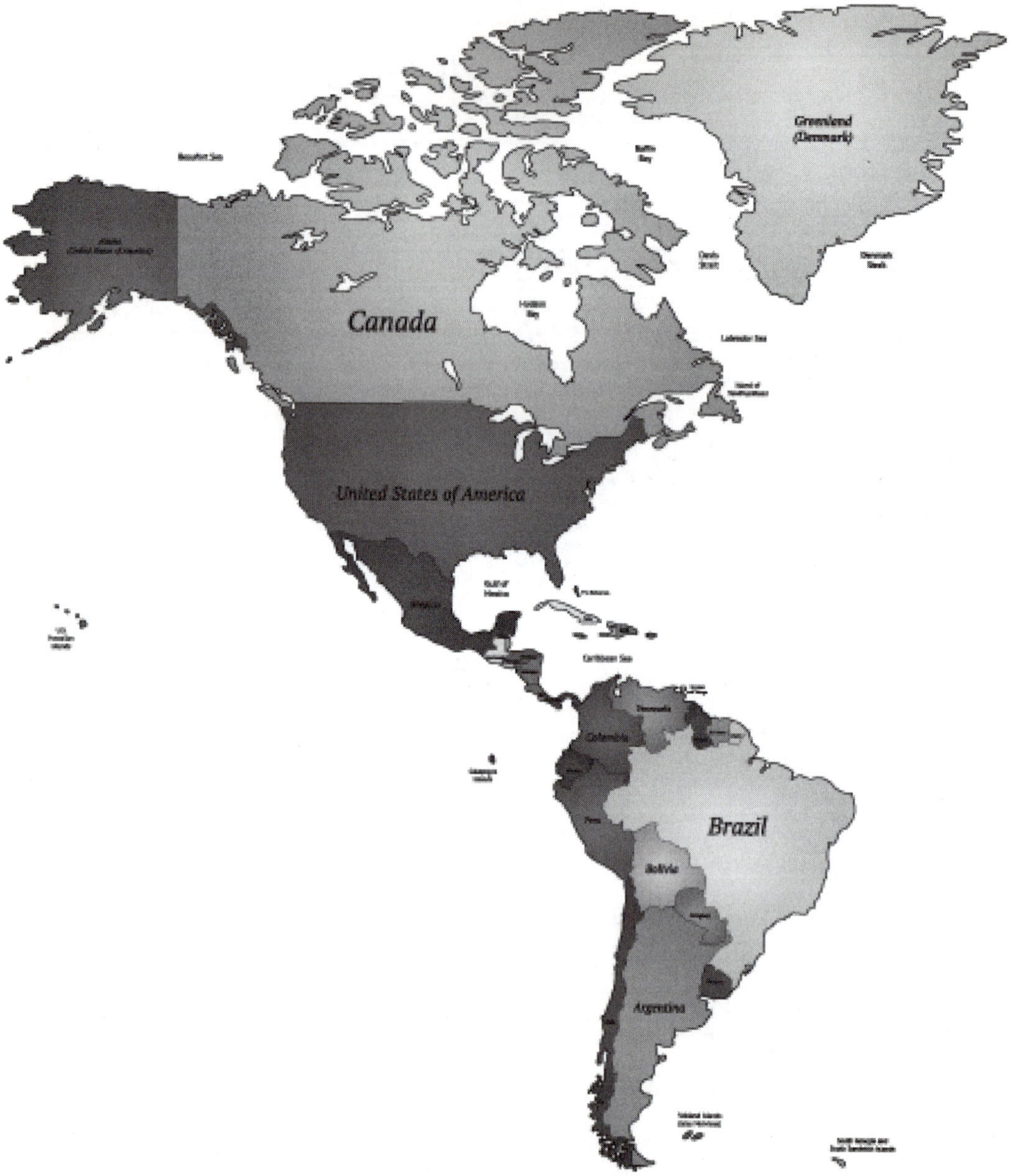

ildogesto / Shutterstock.com

USA and Canada	**Latin America and the Caribbean**
______________________	______________________
______________________	______________________
______________________	______________________
______________________	______________________

(Continued)

Activity C *(Continued)* **Name** ______________________

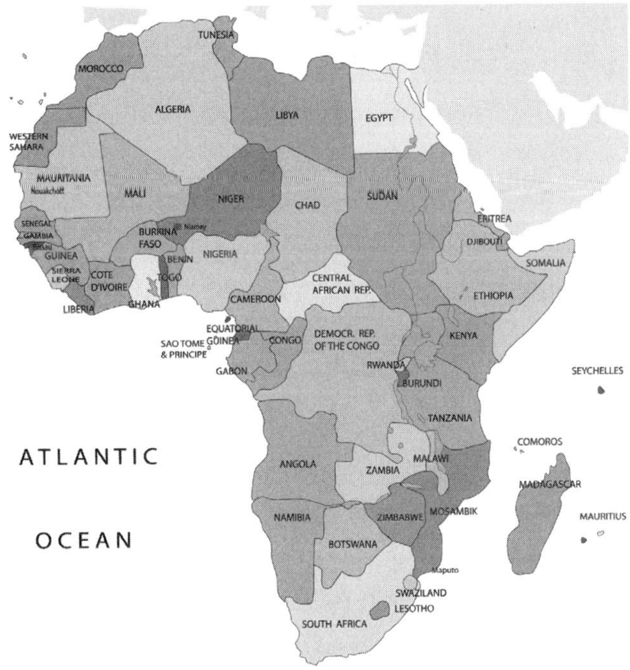

charobnica / Shutterstock.com

Sub-Saharan Africa

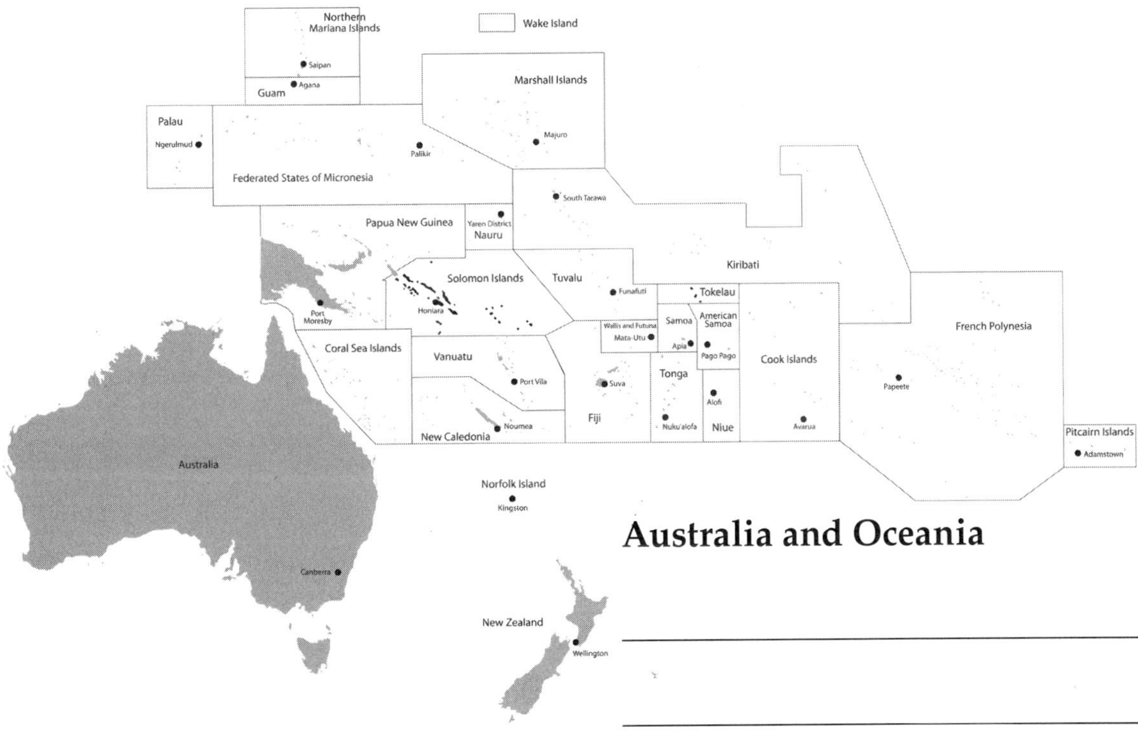

Volina / Shutterstock.com

Australia and Oceania

World Cuisine—Ingredient Matchup

Chapter 52 Name ____________________

Activity D Date __________ Period __________

Match the following terms with the identifying phrases. Terms may be used more than once.

K 1. Potatoes, root vegetables, and cabbages are foundational vegetables in this region.

B 2. In this region, pork is an important meat used in numerous sausages, cured and smoked.

G 3. Salmon, herring, cod, and eels are essential to this region's cuisines.

E 4. Generous use of garlic and herbs is characteristic of this region's cuisine.

F 5. Chicken, lamb, beef, and goat are common meat sources, and yogurt is used in many dishes of this region.

I 6. Ghee, paneer, and yogurt are common dairy products in this region's cuisine.

C 7. The northern tier of this region depends on wheat as a staple ingredient which is used in noodles, dumplings, and pancakes.

J 8. An area of this region is known for its cuisine based on ingredients and cooking styles of African slaves and European planters.

D 9. Native foods of this region include chiles, corn or maize, squashes, beans, amaranth, quinoa, and manioc.

H 10. In this region, wild game—called *bush meat*—supplements domesticated meats and poultry.

A 11. The tropical climate of this region produces an abundance of such fruits as mangoes, coconuts, papaya, bananas, and breadfruit.

H 12. Recipes in this cuisine make great use of rice, millet, sorghum, cassava, yams, black-eyed peas, okra, and peanuts.

A 13. In this region, wild caught, and aquaculture provide such ingredients as salmon, tuna, barramundi, kingfish, pomfret, marlin, mahi-mahi, wahoo, lobster, shrimp, crabs, oysters, and mussels.

A. Australia and Oceania
B. Central and Eastern Europe
C. East Asia
D. Latin America and the Caribbean
E. Mediterranean
F. Middle East and Central Asia
G. Scandinavia
H. Sub-Saharan Africa
I. South Asia
J. USA and Canada
K. Western Europe

(Continued)

Activity D *(Continued)* **Name** ____________________

K 14. Along with the traditionally important sausages and cured meats, dairy products from cows' milk are widely used for cooking, pastries, and cheese-making.

G 15. The mountains and forests of this region provide an abundance of game, wild berries, and mushrooms.

B 16. As well as fresh and fermented cabbage, the cuisine of this region provides such freshwater fish as carp, pike, and perch, and saltwater fish like herring.

E 17. Rice is a staple of this cuisine, and the region's orchards provide oranges, lemons, figs, almonds, and pistachios.

I 18. Chile peppers—often referred to as sambal—are key ingredients in the cuisine of this region.

C 19. The soybean provides nutritious protein in the form of tofu and adds distinct flavors through soy sauce, bean paste, and miso.

D 20. The tropical climate of this region produces its own unique ingredients such as sugarcane, coconut, pineapple, and other tropical fruits.

J 21. The countries of this region are economically developed and have rich agricultural production, plentiful proteins, and extensive coastlines where seafood dominates the cuisine.

H 22. Much of this continent is undeveloped. People make their livelihoods as farmers, herders, and fisherman, which put them close to their food source.

F 23. Historically, this region was part of the spice route from East Asia to Europe. Olive oil, garlic, parsley, and mint add their distinctive flavors to many of the dishes.

I 24. This area is the origin for many of the world's spices, including peppercorns, cloves, ginger, cinnamon, fenugreek, cardamom, nutmeg, and mace.

D 25. The tropical rain forests and jungles of this region provide such exotic cuisine ingredients as acerola, soursop, acaí berries, and Brazil nuts.

Notes

Developing Taste

53

Terminology

Chapter 53

Activity A

Name ______________________

Date __________ Period __________

Below is a professional chef's reply to a student considering a culinary career. Fill in each blank with the appropriate term from Chapter 53. For each term, underline the words in the letter that define that term.

Dear Culinary Hopeful:

You asked about the skills that chefs must develop. Well, of course there are many, and one that you may not have considered is 1.______gustation______, the sense of taste. Did you know that taste involves your nose as well as your mouth? 2.______Olfaction______, or your sense of smell, interprets airborne molecules that enter the nasal cavity and come in contact with the olfactory bulb. The signals travel from the olfactory bulb to the brain for interpretation as "taste." So the nose is important, but it's not the only passage to the olfactory bulb! When you swallow, aromas are 3.______propelled______, or pushed, from the back of your throat up the back of your nasal cavity. This indirect route to the nasal cavity and, ultimately, the olfactory bulb is called the 4. ______retronasal pathway______.

Mouths can actually perceive only five basic tastes. You are probably aware of the basic tastes of sweet, salty, sour, and bitter. There is one more basic taste that Western cultures are just beginning to understand. This taste, called 5. ______umami______, results from a type of protein called a glutamate. It is especially noticeable in fermented soy products, certain ripe vegetables, mushrooms, sea vegetables, aged cheeses, and monosodium glutamate.

Although the mouth can distinguish between only five basic tastes, it can also register the sense of touch. When you chew, the inside of your mouth registers texture. That ability is what allows you to gauge whether a steak is tender or tough. The same ability allows you to perceive 6. ______piquant______, or the spicy hot sensation that is part of some dishes. Foods with chiles, peppercorns, onions, garlic, and mustard produce this sensation.

Developing your sense of taste takes work, but it is well worth the effort. I consider my sense of taste to be the most powerful tool I have for maintaining quality control in the kitchen.

Master Chef

Reviewing Key Concepts

Chapter 53 Name ______________________

Activity B Date __________ Period __________

Circle the clue in parentheses that best completes each of the following statements.

1. The general process of ingesting food is referred to as (**eating**) (**tasting**).
2. (**Eating**) (**Tasting**) requires more concentration than (**eating**) (**tasting**).
3. (**Eating**) (**Tasting**) is the process of thoughtfully analyzing foods and beverages using your senses.
4. Genetic makeup is a (**subjective**) (**physical**) factor that affects taste.
5. Age is a (**subjective**) (**physical**) factor that affects taste.
6. Head trauma and certain medical treatments can be a (**subjective**) (**physical**) factor that affects taste.
7. Memory is a (**subjective**) (**physical**) factor that affects taste.
8. Some medicines are a (**subjective**) (**physical**) factor that affects taste.
9. Culture is a (**subjective**) (**physical**) factor that affects taste.
10. The transmission of aroma molecules to the nasal cavity and olfactory bulb are examples of how the sense of (**smell**) (**taste**) (**touch**) helps our bodies perceive taste.
11. The 10,000 taste buds on the papillae of the tongue are examples of how the sense of (**smell**) (**taste**) (**touch**) helps our bodies perceive taste.
12. The perceived tastes of sweet, salty, sour, bitter, and umami are examples of how the sense of (**smell**) (**taste**) (**touch**) helps our bodies perceive taste.
13. The ability to perceive mustard, chiles, peppercorns, and other piquant ingredients is an example of how the sense of (**smell**) (**taste**) (**touch**) helps our bodies perceive taste.
14. In addition to piquant, the mouth also perceives differences in (**temperature**) (**texture**) (**temperature and texture**).

Taste Combinations

Chapter 53 **Name** ______________________

Activity C **Date** __________ **Period** __________

Part 1

Match the following foods to the taste or sensation they contribute to a dish. Some foods may contribute more than one taste or sensation.

B 1. Chocolate
A 2. Citrus juice
B 3. Coffee
E 4. Honey
E 5. Molasses
F 6. Mushrooms
A, C, D 7. Mustard
F 8. Seaweed
E 9. Sugar
A, E, F 10. Tomato
A 11. Vinegar

A. acid
B. bitter
C. piquant
D. salty
E. sweet
F. umami

Part 2

Complete the basic taste pairings below. **(answers 12–14 can appear in any order)**

12. Sweet and sour
13. Sweet and bitter
14. Sweet and salt
15. Fat and sour
16. Salt and sour

Tasting like a Chef

Chapter 53 **Name** ____________________

Activity D **Date** __________ **Period** __________

Under each of the steps of the *TAAT technique* that follows is a list of statements. If a statement is accurate, place a check mark (✓) in the space provided before each statement.

Step 1: Taste the food.

__✓__ 1. The first step is to see the food, smell it, and place it in your mouth.

______ 2. Serving food to customers without tasting it is an acceptable practice for new cooks.

______ 3. This step is foolish and never occurs in any kitchen.

Step 2: Analyze the food.

______ 4. This step requires little work or concentration.

__✓__ 5. During this step, thought is focused on how the food looks, smells, tastes, and feels.

__✓__ 6. Much concentration is given to the balance of the dish.

__✓__ 7. The chef asks many, many questions during this point.

______ 8. When first learning to taste critically, it is not helpful to write down your impressions and discuss them with others.

Step 3: Adjust the food.

__✓__ 9. Your impressions in Step 2 may make it necessary to adjust the dish.

__✓__ 10. This step may require adding more salt, sugar, or lemon juice.

______ 11. At this step, it is too late for the chef to make the dish more perfect.

Step 4: Taste the food again.

__✓__ 12. Because of adjustments made in Step 3, the process starts over with tasting, analyzing, and adjusting again.

______ 13. It is unusual to need to repeat the process more than one or two times to perfect the dish.

__✓__ 14. The process eventually ends with Step 2 when the chef analyzes the dish and determines it is correct.